Reaching your goal

About the author:

Monika Korber, PhD; MA, BA psychotherapy science Mediator and psychotherapist, systemic familientherapy, life- and social counsellor; lecturer at Sigmund Freud University, SFU Vienna; lecturer at other institutes such as University Institute ARGE Bildungsmanagement; Mediation Training Institute I.A.M.S.; Experience in practice, teaching and research (non exhaustive list): Private practice in Vienna and in Lower Austria; Coaching in organizations and companies; Participation in inter-ministerial working groups

Previously: *BEST* Personality Training; Head of a child protection center; Child and Youth Ombudsoffice in Vienna; Initiative and implementation of professional mediation in schools in several districts in Vienna within the Kinder- und Jugendanwaltschaft – Project turned into association „*together*" – founding member;
Expert opinions for the Austrian Health Ministry; International working experience (research, psychosocial field, tourism) in India, Europe, etc.

contact: mkorber@joeya.net

Translation:
Jenny Baer-Pásztory
www.baerconsulting.eu/translation

MONIKA KORBER

Reaching your goal

Social Business –
How dreams are turned into start-ups

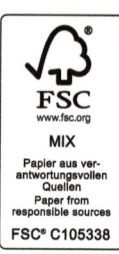

Bibliographical Information of the Deutsche Nationalbibliothek

This publication is listed in the
Deutsche Nationalbibliographie
of the Deutsche Nationalbibliothek;
detailed bibliographical information
can be accessed under http: //dnb.d-nb.de

Printing, Production and Layout: BoD – Books on Demand
ISBN: 978-3-7448-6151-9

Content

Foreword

Reaching your goal

What can I say about this book, other than that - apart from it being a very interesting topic *per* se, it is extremely interesting due to the profound expertise which Dr. Monika Korber has acquired throughout her many years of working as a professional.

Monika Korber's knowledge of social business was deepened by the conversations she had with key social entrepreneurs throughout the world. In writing this book she is now passing on this knowledge to others. It will be most helpful to all those who want to fulfill their own professional and existential dreams, too, also with the aid of this book.

This book is special, bearing in mind that she did not study the world of social business merely to be able to write a book about it. Monika Korber's focus has always been helping others. It comes as no surprise that she chose a profession in the areas of health and social affairs which she pursues with more than average commitment and competence. Most of those who have had the pleasure of meeting her and who have benefited from her work, be it clients, students, colleagues, family members and friends can testify this. Myself, I have had the opportunity to be convinced by her professional devotion over the years that she is a trainer at the International Archaic and Modern School (I.A.M.S.), my training institute which has been certified by the Austrian Ministry of Justice and the Chamber of Commerce.

I warmly welcome you to read this book which has the potential to help you change your life.

Angelantonio Ferrandina

Director of I.A.M.S.
Registered Mediator
Social and Life Counsellor
LifeCoach, Artist
email: iams@trilogis.at

Dedication

To all positive people.

Acknowledgements

Sincere appreciation to **ALL** of you who contributed directly or indirectly to this book, some amongst them are listed here: Ravi Agarwal, Jenny Baer-Pásztory, Jeroo Billimoria, Bill Drayton, Thomas Druyen, Jutta Fiegl, Patricia Kahane, Michael Kierein, Judy Korn, Kathrin Mörtl, Heinz Laubreuter, Rebecca Onie, Earl Martin Phalen, Alfred Pritz, Johannes Reichmayr, Bernd Rieken, Marco Roveda, Gloria de Souza, Alisa del Tufo, Götz Werner, Muhammad Yunus.

Heartfelt thanks to my family and to all my friends who have supported me in their individual ways and measure.

And my deep gratitude goes to my LifeCoach who's contributions have been invaluable to the content and in the realization of this oeuvre.

Introduction

How do social entrepreneurs feel, think and act and what are the ingredients for their success?[1]

This is the central theme of this book which is based on the results of a scientific study I undertook.[2] Helpful factors and mental patterns which have supported the sustainable success of the social entrepreneurs I spoke to are described. The psychotherapy sciences are especially suited to try to find answers to subjective complexe matters. My practical experience as a psychotherapist, counsellor and mediator helped me to gain insights.

On a general note psychotherapy can help people change their attitude and behaviour so that they suffer less.[3] They feel better understood and learn how to deal with other people and situations more constructively. As a consequence their suffering and illness can be reduced and health and wellbeing can increase, making them more able to meet their individual challenges.

Generally psychotherapy can help to create a more humane environment. It contributes to constructive changes in society such as helping us meet the challenges of our time with focus and courage, such as in social business. This publication sheds light on some of the extraordinary personalities of the rapidly growing third sector,[4] the economic sector which is non-governmental and not primarily profit orientated.[5] Other terms used for it are the non-profit sector, the civilian sector as well as parts of the charity sector.

The book tries to illustrate some of the inner structures of social entrepreneurs combined with socio-cultural and scientific aspects. The findings are based on personal conversations I had with social entrepreneurs in various parts of the world. All of them have realized their ideas and visions and turned them into success. They have managed to find solutions to a number of problems faced by millions of people. These problems relate to a variety of areas, including the health and education system, prevention of domestic violence and the environment. They speak of an enormous transition which is underway, for instance how much a paradigm change has become necessary in education and training. Marco Roveda, a social entrepreneur who works in the environmental area uses drastic words: "People need to change if they want to survive."[6]

Some elements of the success of these personalities can serve as guiding principles. An increase in the awareness of social business might encourage people to try to make their own dreams and ideas come true. This was one of the reasons I wanted to write this book. All over the world social entrepreneurs go new ways, develop new models and take on social responsibility. This is a particular issue in the professional environment which is becoming tougher and tougher for many. I would therefore like to briefly take a psychotherapeutic view on this part of our life.

Work and Mental Pressure

Working conditions can lead to a deterioration of our health, both physically and mentally. One of the underlying causes for why work environments can be damaging is that often the main focus is on profit maximization. Most work practices are geared towards this focus, often ignoring other values. The individual and collective exploitation of people, resources and our planet are the consequences. Human beings and the natural environment are doomed to pay the price.

Mental health problems caused by pressures at the workplace are on the rise. There are many symptoms, including various types of anxiety, depression, sleep disorders and burn-out.[7] Since 2013, Austrian companies are duty bound to examine workplaces with regard to mental pressures. Another important achievement of some of the Austrian federal provinces is access to psychotherapy financed by public health insurance, but still a lot remains to be done. In the public health sector Austria set a milestone with its Psychotherapy Act in 1990. Internationally it can be considered best practice.[8]

A team of psychologists and psychotherapists working with Wittchen estimated the annual costs of the inability to work and of impaired social relationships as hundreds of billions of Euros. The most frequent symptoms are depression, sleep and anxiety disorders. When comparing the results of the various countries no significant cultural or national differences were found. The study showed that, already today, mental and neurological illnesses represent the highest cost factor in Europe.[9]

Reasons for the disorders are quoted as pressure to perform, mobbing and a lack of acknowledgement, to mention just a few and many issues related to the ever increasing presence of the digital world. Some health insurance providers now focus on mental illness prevention within companies. A positive example of prevention is the European campaign "Work. In tune with life. Move Europe."

The authors of the EU study consider mental disorders the largest challenge for European health policies in the 21st century. The economic losses which companies suffer through the amount of sick leave taken due to mental disorders plus inefficient working hours is enormous.[10] According to a report by WIFO, the Austrian Institute of Economic Research in Vienna, the damage to the Austrian economy caused by non-treatment of mental disorders is approximately 2.8 billion Euros a year. Here future-orientated and responsible actions by those in charge are called for. Decisions urgently need to be made to reduce the enormous economic damage caused by health problems including mental health. Those responsible may have the chance to demonstrate sustainability and vision as well, but they will certainly achieve cost efficiency in any case.[11] Within only a short period of time the benefits would be quantifiable. In his book "Happy Princes"[12] Thomas Druyen argues that health should be defined as wealth. Druyen sees the prevention of illness as a constructive element of the culture of wealth. "The conscious preservation of health is not only a rational necessity, but also an ethical responsibility towards the community".

He also states that

"the culture of wealth is based on the conviction that every human being has the duty to use his or her wealth beneficially. If we truly lived our culture of wealth, this would add value to the way we deal with ourselves and with others."

Every wage earner remembers situations where she or he was not able to work as efficiently as usual, was not able to perform as well due to psychological pressures e.g. family trouble, problems in relationships or psychosomatic problems. And this is without being diagnosed as being mentally ill. In case of mental illness the reduction in work performance is even more pronounced.

A central task of psychotherapy is to contribute to "... reducing or removing existing symptoms, changing disturbed behavior and attitudes and supporting maturation, development and health."[13]

Mentally healthy human beings recognize their own capabilities and can make use of them. Some of these people could become social entrepreneurs, employing these capabilities for common welfare and contributing towards solutions to problems in our society.

What is a Social Entrepreneur?

Over the past few years the terms "social entrepreneur" and "social business" have become quite familiar in the German-speaking countries.[14] In the English-speaking part of the world, they have become the "big words in town".

There is no single definition for "social entrepreneurs". The various definitions, which different authors use, reflect their self perception and world view and the individual scientific approach they follow. For instance Achleitner and her co-authors use a broad definition. "A social entrepreneur is a person whose prime aim it is to find a solution to a social problem by applying entrepreneurial tools."[15]

Entrepreneurial activity to try and solve social problems has been known throughout history. It took various forms and was given various names. Many state-run, confessional and other institutions, which are now taken for granted in modern and post-modern societies, were initiated by social entrepreneurs such as Hermann Gmeiner (SOS Children's Villages (SOS Kinderdörfer), Maria Montessori (education, schools) and many others. The phenomenon of the social entrepreneur is not new.

Concepts of social business are becoming more and more attractive. Over the past few years the third sector,[16] the non-profit public welfare sector, has received more and more attention in Germany and Austria. So what is the spirit of social entrepreneurship? Thomas Druyen describes it as follows:

"the ability to act entrepreneurially and charitably at the same time, to bundle activities, to create synergies or open up new knowledge, to recognize societal inequalities and reduce them efficiently."[17]

Rigid economic and societal thinking patterns have long been challenged by critics and pioneers. The economic crisis in 2008 with all its consequences confirm that they are right. We are in the midst of an enormous global transition characterized by societal, ecological, economic and political processes. Social entrepreneurs and their impact on society are important players in this process. However, this certainly does not imply that the state can shrug off its responsibility. This is often used as an argument against social entrepreneurship by its critics. By following its vision, social business has enabled millions of people to lead a more humane existence with a higher standard of living. A leading example globally is Professor Muhammad Yunus who was awarded the Nobel Peace Prize in 2006. Starting off in Bangladesh he developed a system of microcredits which helps many poor people to survive, to enjoy work and to develop personally.

In this book the English terms "social enterprise" and "social business" are treated as synonyms. David Bornstein's translated publication "How to Change the World: Social Entrepreneurs and the Power of New Ideas" helped to introduce the term "social entrepreneur" into the German language.[18]

Although other concepts such as "Corporate-Social-Responsibility" (CSR) contain the word "social", many of them do not take the social aspect too seriously. Companies with CSR-departments call themselves "social businesses" in the hope that this may give them a competitive advantage. Profit maximization remains the prime aim for many. They are only marginally interested in tackling social problems when supporting a social project.[19]

The term "entrepreneur" is derived from the French where it has been known since the 17th and 18th century. An "entrepreneur" is someone who does something, who becomes active. The French economist Baptiste Say gave the term its specific meaning around the turn of the 19th century: a person who supports economic progress by a project or activity which finds new and better ways.[20] Years ago the combination of the terms "entrepreneur" and "social" would have seemed contradictory in many countries, despite several historical examples which illustrate that this combination is indeed possible (e.g. hospice care).

J. Gregory Dees, director of the Centre for the Advancement of Social Entrepreneurship at Duke University's Fuqua School of Business, defines the social entrepreneur as a business person with a social mission. In his article "The Meaning of Social Entrepreneurship" he combines models from the research on entrepreneurship.[21] He includes Jean Baptiste Say's theory of added value, Joseph Schumpeter's theory of the change agents, Peter Drucker's thoughts on the search for opportunities and those on "resourcefulness" by Howard Stevenson.[22] Dees summarizes the role of social entrepreneurs as "change agents" as follows:[23]

- "adopting a mission to create and sustain social value (not just private value);
- recognizing and relentlessly pursuing new opportunities to serve that mission;
- engaging in a process of continuous innovation, adaptation, and learning;
- acting boldly without being limited by resources currently in hand; and
- exhibiting heightened accountability to the constituencies served and for the outcomes created."

It is an idealized definition. Its criteria are met in a host of different ways by the social entrepreneurs I spoke to. According to Dees, the more completely a person fulfills the above criteria, the more she or he fits into the model of the social entrepreneur. But to gain a deeper understanding of social entrepreneurship, he suggests that the ideas of the authors above should be used for additional orientation, as, in a world of frequently blurred boundaries, some of the criteria might in fact be applicable to both business and social business alike.[24]

According to Bill Drayton, the founder of Ashoka (the global association of social entrepreneurs), social entrepreneurs are people whose holistic business approach helps to find sustainable solutions to a number of problems. They are passionate and have high ethical values. Ashoka has developed a way to identify such people.[25] Drayton speaks about social entrepreneurs as "men and women with system changing solutions for the most pressing social challenges of our world."[26] He was one of the driving forces in coining the term "social entrepreneur" and making it known. Some of Bill Drayton's statements and insights from the interview he gave me are included in this book. Drayton defines the following selection criteria for Ashoka fellows. They must have

- a new idea to solve a critical social problem
- high ethical standards
- an entrepreneurial personality
- high creativity and
- the vision of an extensive social impact of this idea.[27]

The psychotherapist Ryzard Praszkier and his co-authors similarly describe social entrepreneursas passionate, ethical individuals who solve large social problems using new approaches.[28] The social scientists and economists Johanna Mair, Ignasi Martí as well as Roger L. Martin und Sally Osberg reflect extensively on the definition of social entrepreneurship.[29] They quote the following components, amongst others:[30]

- the identification of a condition which causes human suffering and which cannot be overcome by the affected group itself;
- taking action to improve this condition substantially within society - for the affected group and
- for oneself.[31]

Muhammad Yunus is one of the most prominent pioneers of social business and one of the interview partners of my study. Through his ground-breaking system of microcredits Yunus proves that inhumane business habits can be changed fundamentally for the benefit of the poor and disadvantaged. His model of microfinancing is being emulated globally and enables the poor to take advantage of bank credits. Thanks to him, social business has received large momentum globally.[32] Yunus distinguishes two types of social business: in the first type the focus lies on the benefits for society, such as enabling access to food, housing, education, health care and prevention of violence, instead of maximizing profits for the owners of a company. In the second type the poor become actual shareholders of the company. In this case the social benefit is seen in their corporate ownership. The management of the company establishes transparent criteria for the classification of poverty.[33]

The difference between the social business person and the business person is the way he or she uses the profits – either primarily to invest in ways which benefit society or else primarily to serve his or her own benefits.

Martin and Osberg argue that straightforward entrepreneurs, too, are also often not motivated by the expectation of financial profit either. What motivates them makes the difference, but also what the profits are used for. Seen from an ethical perspective, it certainly makes a difference whether profits are used for personal benefits or whether they are invested primarily to improve common welfare. To quote the social scientist Gregory Bateson[34] 'it is the difference which makes a difference'.

Yunus's social business model of microcredits serves as an example to illustrate this. The bank he founded, the Grameenbank and the various social businesses which have arisen from it are designed to make a profit. This profit is reinvested into the bank and its projects with the aim of providing more and more people with the necessary help and support to improve their quality of life. Profits are not used for personal benefits.

Finally my definition of the term "social entrepreneur". It is a pragmatic one, which leans towards that of Ashoka. The main focus of the social entrepreneur is the social concern. Key for him or her is to deal with social problems and achieve a change of the undesirable situation. So:

"A social entrepreneur is a personality who is aware of urgent problems of those who cannot solve these problems themselves. She or he will take action responsibly and join forces with others in facing these challenges locally and in the wider context and finding sustainable solutions using creative, entrepreneurial approaches. The entrepreneurial approach is a means to reach this aim."

The following chapters approach the complex topic of how do personalities who have managed to realize their visions and dreams feel, think and act by having a look at some of the ingredients for the success of social entrepreneurs.

2. Core Motivations

What motivates continuously successful social entrepreneurs and which factors have helped them is illustrated in this chapter. The insights were gained, amongst others, by a psychotherapeutic scientific study which forms the basis of this book.[35]

The main aim of the study was to find out which elements are helpful to social entrepreneurs in implementing their social ideas, dreams and projects.

2.1 Formative experiences

This chapter describes some of the formative experiences of social entrepreneurs which influenced their decision to become one. They speak of experiences which touched them deeply emotionally and which motivated them to take action.

They describe deep emotional experiences in one or several phases of their lives (childhood, adolescence, adulthood) which left a mark and which became an important incentive for what they do. The formative experiences include both positive and burdening ones. Both produced strong emotions including anger, shock, grief, surprise or joy.

Prof. Muhammad Yunus describes formative experiences in his daily confrontation with people who were dying of hunger – right in front of the university where he lectured. He felt the strong need to do something, to become active. This personal confrontation shook him to the core. He described how he saw how close life and death were to each other. Side by side. It was often difficult to distinguish whether mother and child were still alive or not. It became impossible for him to continue teaching his students economic theories, explaining to them how economy works, whilst people were dying right in front of the university. They were dying, simply because they did not have enough to eat. He felt the urgent wish to help, to be of use somehow and started to get into motion.[36]

"I wanted to see if I can be of some help to one individual, just one individual. So I was not thinking about the whole country, all the problems, just help one person. I don't know what that help would be, I said, as a human being I can stand next to another human being and offer myself to help him or help her in any way I can."[37]

The next example illustrates how an emotionally positive formative experience lead the social engagement of Gloria de Souza in a certain direction. She saw how creative and effective learning can work for children in India. She was visiting a workshop where great new learning methods were being demonstrated. *Children learnt via experience.* "I really felt, yes, this is what education should be like and why does it have to start so late?"[38] (Note: as the workshop was targeted towards older children).

And:

"My goodness, this is something, that is showing us how good learning can actually take place, how effective learning for every child can take place! So I was finding an answer to all the questions that I had."[39]

A difficult experience plus the emotions it triggers can also lead to the unfolding of potential, to intensified activity. The following citations illustrate this. They also show how far-reaching the effects of the decision of a single person to do something beneficial can be.

"I discovered by chance, that the forest is going to be cut down and be given to developing agencies and I felt this was wrong. I had no idea of what to do, but I decided to do something about it, just as a citizen."

"I was angry. I have this deep relationship with nature, the idea of nature. I feel really, if somebody is cutting a tree, I feel agitated inside. If somebody is doing something which is I think, unjust, unfair, I get agitated inside. I feel this is not right. And then I need to do something about it."[40]

The forest referred to is a huge area surrounding the town of Delhi in India, a metropolis of over 16 million inhabitants. The forest exists to this day due to the commitment at the time of Ravi Agarwal, a social entrepreneur and artist. Meanwhile the forest is protected by law and continues to increase the quality of life for millions of people.

The social entrepreneur Bill Drayton remembers that his social commitment started early, in elementary school.

One of his formative experiences was a typewritten newspaper which he made a great effort to produce for all his classmates. Although it was a lot of work at the time he felt it was important that everybody in class should receive a copy. A further formative experience was when he first met his uncle from Australia. It left a lasting impression on him. His uncle had contracted polio at age three, but had still managed to work his way up to becoming a judge at the Supreme Court. Drayton felt as though he was meeting himself, as he shared so many values with him.[41]

Another social entrepreneur had experienced at close range how her grandmother had cared for the aged and sick and had helped people in need. As a small child she had experienced how it feels to help.

Some social entrepreneurs suffered large personal losses due to the sudden death of people close to them. The death of a beloved person is a profound experience and can become a *change agent*. This fact is also of relevance in psychotherapy. A person can, even as a child, develop positive things for his or her life from emotionally burdening or even traumatic experiences. However, this does not mean that this is possible for everyone or that challenging circumstances or traumatic experiences should be seen as positive per se. Also this shall in no way lead to a trivialization or a playing down of the individual suffering experienced.

A formative experience for another social entrepreneur was the fact that, as a child, he was discriminated against by other children. This caused him a lot of pain. He managed to develop strength from this experience. He committed himself to seeing that others did not have to go through the same pain. As a young adult he made a decision:

"I just decided, I didn't want other people to feel the way I felt in that moment. [...] I said, let's get involved in politics and help out-groups, because it seems that there are more out-groups than there are in-groups."[42]

During a placement, Earl Martin Phalen, social entrepreneur and founder of Summeradvantage, asked a small child a mathematical question. An older child jumped in and answered the question perfectly for it. He quoted this as a formative experience for him.

"[...] her eyes lit up and I just felt, this is what I am called to do. I knew from that moment that I was going into education and this is my purpose [...] I really feel fortunate to know to have had such clarity [...] those were the things that you lean on when things get hard and you start having challenges of: 'can you do this?'"[43]

Another social entrepreneur describes painful family experiences when his siblings died. Very early on he was confronted with the death of people close to him. His mother fell ill, too, and although the family made every effort, no effective help could be found for her. At an early age he experienced difficult situations and had to take on a lot of responsibility such as caring for his younger siblings. Viewed therapeutically, parentification can arise in such a situation, meaning that children take on responsibilities of the parent. Resilient children, however, can develop positive aspects from this. He started to practice reframing as a child and began to evaluate a burdening experience in a different way. Reframing means to give the event a new reference framework. In an autobiography he describes this as a game he used to play with his brother. They undertook a kind of "weather forecast" for the day, referring to the state of the ill family member. "What is the forecast for today?"[44] Existential experiences and being able to deal with them with the necessary creativity and flexibility can be encouraging on the one hand, but can also reduce fear. Faced with death, many other problems in life become relative. Heavy experiences can support the desire and the commitment to help people in need.

Social entrepreneur Alisa del Tufo told the story of how, during her work for the prevention of domestic violence, she was shocked to find out that a child had been murdered by its father. Although he had been beating the mother for a long time, the mother had never turned to a help centre.

"[…] a murder of a little girl […] I was very upset by the fact that as a domestic violence organization we weren't really thinking very much about the children. I was very upset that here was a woman who had been beaten for so long and she'd never been in one of the domestic violence programs. I started talking to the women who were coming to sanctuary, I started hearing, I wanted to understand this much more deeply and I wanted to change the way the domestic violence and the way the child welfare movement worked, because they were like silos, they where two independent rivers, that weren't connected at all."[45]

She transformed these profound experiences into additional social dedication to people in crisis.[46] Alisa del Tufo changed the way programmes on the prevention of domestic violence worked at the time in the US by connecting them with the movement of child protection.

The following experience left a lasting impression on Judy Korn: she experienced a confrontation between a group of left and a group of right wing youths. They were political enemies, the situation was escalating and a physical fight was about to start. Korn felt that violence was no solution. It would only make things worse. So she and a friend stood up and she asked those who were about to use their fists why they were doing this.

"[...] and then I gathered all my courage and simply walked over to this group of right-wing youths with my school friend and asked them why they were doing this. [...] Mercilessly naïve, but, anyway, this is what we did. We completely threw them with our naivety. It worked. This was the start of a project between this right-wing group and the students which belonged more to the left wing politically and the whole scene calmed down."[47]

This courageous intervention managed to break down hardened prejudices within a very short period of time by inviting communication between both groups. Rather than ending in violence, the conflict ended peacefully.

Judy Korn's courage made her realize that it is worth approaching opponents, even though they may have completely opposite views. It is worthwhile asking them what drives them. Encouraged by this formative experience she decided later to work with juvenile delinquents and developed methods for the prevention of violence.

Several of the interviewees managed to develop enormous potential, sometimes even in their early childhood, despite deeply unsettling experiences.

Research on resilience focuses on precisely these resources of a person. Emmy Werner and Ruth Smith state that resilience can even develop, in crises, if these crisis are managed successfully. They demonstrated that the development of resilience and protective factors, which help people adapt to a difficult situation constructively, can continue throughout a lifetime. Resilience develops in response to having to cope with challenges and crises.[48]

Systemic psychotherapy, too, aims at building upon the available resources of a person. Dysfunctions receive the necessary attention, but no more than is needed. The psychotherapist Gunter Schmid illustrates this with a sense of humour. In his seminars he sometimes tells the participants things like: so far you have managed to survive all these difficult and terrible things. You must have incredible resources to be able to do so. You will not easily be thrown off track anymore.[49]

Social entrepreneurs frequently transformed crises or difficult experiences of their childhood into helpful personal resources. Some popular theories still maintain that the personality of a person is formed mainly during the first three years of his or her life, that their education and environment are their main influences and that these early formative years determine who they are. Jens Asendorpf, psychologist of the Humboldt University in Berlin who has been working on the complexities of the personality for many years, stated during an interview:

"Meanwhile it has been disproven that the human personality is formed and becomes consolidated mainly during the first years of a person's life [...] Early childhood is not that formative and influential at all. It is not responsible for the great variation in the normal scope of personality. Classic attachment theory puts too much value on this aspect."[50]

This puts the deterministic factor back into perspective. Some psychological and psychotherapeutic disciplines have the tendency to interpret stressful experiences of childhood exclusively from the point of view of deficits. This contradicts the insights of the research on resilience. Further, the principle of hope plays an important role in reducing suffering and supporting health.

The formative experiences, which the interviewees describe, illustrate how both positive and challenging experiences were key influences which supported their development as social entrepreneurs (ESSE).

2.2 Questions of Meaning

The question of meaning of what they do is fundamental for social entrepreneurs. "Where do I belong?" "What am I doing here, is this the right thing to do?"[51] They ask themselves these and other similar questions and reflect on existential issues such as finding their own place in life. These essential questions lead them to making decisions which are sometimes radical. They change their lives and create something which makes sense to them and gives meaning to their lives. Ravi Agarwal does the work also because he feels happy doing it. It makes him feel part of this world. This work is what he can do without personal conflict. He describes this as follows:

"For me it is like finding my own place like where I belong and I don't think one completely finds it ever, in the world outside. I get more and more focused on what I really want to do in my life."[52]

In Alisa del Tufo's words. "[...] and I began to really think about my role in the world and how could I be a part of the solution rather than part of the problem."[53]

The social entrepreneur Earl Martin Phalen remembers his experience of when he saw just how much joy education can give children. This was a key moment for him which convinced him of his vocation: to get into education himself: "I felt it and knew, every vibe was like this is why I am here, this is my purpose in life."[54]

A motivation for doing what they do often stems from reflecting on the meaning of their lives. This aspect can also be seen in Muhammad Yunus's words: "The only thing I wanted, to help, I wanted to be of some use, use me I'm here."[55]

Gloria de Souza describes her vision of the meaning of life as follows:

"For me there is a vision and that vision is, that human beings in the universe for that matter have been created to really enjoy their strength, every bit of what they are able to do and achieve and we are here to help each other, realize our potential. My vision is, that life must become beautiful for all of us and if I somehow become part of this world of being able to educate, so I'm trying to draw out the best of that." "I love what I am doing, there are so many moments of joy, that you would never know I experience, which keeps me there. This is my reason for living. I don't think I need to be good, because I am waiting for a reward, honour. No, so whether there is a reward or punishment, that doesn't mean anything to me, but what I do want to experience, this life is the joy of goodness to be shared and that is heaven for me."[56]

For some people doing what has meaning makes them feel happy. This includes Jeroo Billimoria, a serial social entrepreneur who also founded the child helpline in India and Aflatoun International: "I think, people must do what they feel happy doing, that's my only thing. I am happy doing what I do. What more do you want in life?"[57]

The social entrepreneur Marco Roveda founder and president of Lifegate[58] emphasises that being happy gives his life meaning. It is his personal fulfillment. He became aware of that when his former formula of "study, work, earn money" no longer satisfied him. He noticed that although it provided him with a comfortable life, it did not make him happy. So he stopped. He terminated his former career, closed both his businesses and embarked on his quest for happiness and meaning in his life. He realized that being happy is completely intangible, has nothing to do with material goods. A formula based on material values would not be able to create an intangible result. His search was successful. The basis of all this values for him is *the Good*. On his quest for happiness which represents the meaning of life he identified the following values:

"Living sensitively, finding meaning for my life, being aware of how and what I consume, respecting the ecosystem and all forms of life, looking for work which satisfies me, being honest with myself and with others, doing good, choosing true friends, letting go of pain, fear and anger and living life joyfully. These are my values." And: " I started to lead my life according to these values. They directed me to starting up an agricultural project called Scaldasole which provided the foundation for the organic market in Italy. We spread the concept of respect for the environment and respect for people with our organic products."[59]

The founder of *dm* (a health and beauty retailer, drugstore) and lecturer on social business Götz Werner describes his motivation and inner attitude as follows:

"If you see meaning in something you can motivate yourself intrinsically. [...] A person who is intrinsically motivated will find ways. A person who is not will always finds reasons. That's the point. And this is so on all levels, on the personal level, the private level, on the family level in companies and in the entire economy."[60]

Social entrepreneurs rate their immaterial wishes higher than material ones. They turn down well paid job offers to pursue activities which have meaning for them and which help them follow their vision. Their priority is not to have a comfortable life, money, possessions and status.

Professor Muhammad Yunus is another good example. He quit his work as a well respected professor at a university to help the poor, as this is what he felt had more meaning. Others close their own businesses, even though they may be profitable, or they take the decision not to go down the typical business career path at all and choose to help people in need or the environment instead.[61] It gives their life meaning and fulfills them. They do not regret the life-changing decisions they have to make to be able to follow their calling as a social entrepreneur, even though some of them can be very hard. One of the social entrepreneurs denied himself the pleasure of being with his first child to be able to pursue his social activities. He had to make this difficult choice when his partner returned to her country of origin to raise the child there and his work prevented him from joining them.

As the work is meaningful, it is done with joy. "I love what I am doing", Gloria de Souza says about her work with children in the area of environmental education.[62] Many bring incredible enthusiasm into their work.

The question of meaning is core to social business personalities. A fundamental value is the desire to help others. In his autobiography, Muhammad Yunus writes that he felt empty and thought the economic theories which he was lecturing about at university were meaningless in the face of the many people which were starving to death. He needed to find out whether he could be useful to others in some way, whether he could help. So he left his prestigious role of a professor and started talking to people in a nearby village. Not as an expert, but as someone who wanted to learn. He wanted to understand how he could help them. His activities started to develop meaning.[63] Ravi Agarwal, does "performance work". He reflects: "Who am I, what is my role, what is my responsibility [...] And getting to know my own self and the self of others, this is what I am really interested in." [64]

Here are some of the most concise quotes of some of the social entrepreneurs when speaking about the meaning of their existence and their work (see also their websites):

"I love what I am doing, [...] there are so many moments of joy, that you would never know, I experience, which keeps me there. This is my reason for living." (Gloria de Souza)

"I began to really think about my role in the world and how could I be a part of the solution rather than part of the problem."(Alisa del Tufo)

"I realized that to be happy my life had to have meaning. We have to do good."[65](Marco Roveda)

"If you see meaning in something, you can motivate yourself intrinsically."(Götz Werner)

"And I knew, every vibe was like this is why I am here, this is my purpose in life." (Earl Martin Phalen)

Following certain profound experiences, the question of meaning becomes essential for some social entrepreneurs. It gives them even more clarity in their purpose in life and even more joy in realizing their vision. Social entrepreneurs want to effect something. Some also see what they do as their vocation. In Earl Martin Phalen's words:

"Once I found my calling, there was no way that I was gonna waste my life. Tomorrow is not granted, so I wasn't to waste my life doing something for 20 years and then coming back later to my passion or spending 80 to 100 hours a week doing something to pay the bills and then on my free time do the thing I was passionate about, there was no way I was gonna do that."[66]

Viktor Frankl, an Austrian neurologist and psychotherapist, survived four Nazi concentration camps. His wife, his parents and his brother did not. Frankl founded the psychotherapeutic school of existential analysis and logo-therapy and worked intensely on the question of sense and meaning. He often quoted Nietzsche's saying: "He who has a why to live can bear almost any how."[67] He recognized the existential relevance of sense in a person's life. How it strengthens a person's will and psyche. He found his own meaning in life in helping others to find theirs. For Frankl the core issue of logotherapy was "the self determination of a person based on his or her sense of responsibility and his or her definition of meaning and personal set of values".[68]

Another Austrian psychotherapist, Alfried Längle, reported on a survey which was undertaken in Vienna in 2000 on the topic of *sense*[69] The survey results showed that 96% of the people who took part had frequently asked themselves what meaning their life had. However, people usually only think about this crucial question consciously when they find themselves in a difficult situation. Indeed the survey showed that people leading a satisfying, fulfilling and meaningful life ask themselves this question less often.

A further element of the success of the interview partners is the realization that they have profited personally in a non-material way by finding meaning in what they do. Each one of them is well aware of this. One of them says: "It's a blessing to be able to live your life in service to your personal mission."[70] This and similar statements disprove the argument which is sometimes used by critics that social entrepreneurs do not reflect on their own psyche.

Dominique Debats[71] examined what effect seeing meaning in one's life has. He found that people who see a meaning in their life suffer less from mental stress, have more confidence and are happier than people who do not.

The research focus of Matthias Beck, medical specialist and theologist at the University of Vienna, is an interdisciplinary view on the relationship of body and soul. He found that gradually biologists, too, are rethinking. The body is no longer seen as an isolated mechanistic structure which can be repaired if necessary. The human body, its health and questions about the meaning of life are interconnected.[72]

Bernd Rieken states that the individual quest for meaning was not needed in earlier societies, as then people defined themselves primarily via parameters of collective socialisation. [73] Nowadays this individual quest has become much more important, particular in western, more individualistic societies. It is a demanding task which all the interview partners have taken on.

The tireless engagement of the social entrepreneurs and the joy and satisfaction associated with it is based, too, on the meaningfulness of what they do (ESSE). They live a life which is, for them, filled with meaning. The majority of the interviewees connect this with a spiritual dimension which forms a firm part of their lives.

2.3 The Good as the Reason for Action

Social entrepreneurs aim at achieving positive things for other people and/or the environment. At the same time they turn their concept of what is good into reality. They invest a lot of energy and courage explicitly to help other people or to bring about changes to support the protection of the environment. This commitment is paired with a strong sense of justice. They become active for a liveable environment, for the poor, for education, for people in crises, for those who are ill and those in need. Bill Drayton, founder of the global network Ashoka, sums it up as follows: "That's what defines the field. It is being for the good, that is the purpose."[74] To do good is an important value for social entrepreneurs. Thomas Druyen's thoughts on this in his book "Happy Princes" are as follows:

"We provide the unfathomless of our psyche with contours by adopting a framework of reliable values. With our personal talents and cultural conditions we form that personality which leads us more and more out of immaturity. This claim of being able to shape oneself is not an utopian dream. Millions of social entrepreneurs demonstrate daily how they manage to transform the power of new ideas."[75]

Ravi Agarwal described how it churns him up inside if he sees injustice and how he feels compelled to act. Social entrepreneurs support humanity, being there for each other and learning from each other. They are interested in the development of potentials. In Gloria de Souza's words:

"We have all our own individual Self so wonderfully unique each one. But I cannot be that special Self even, unless I am acknowledging that we need each other. So that vital message is a great one for believing human beings who see, I'm very special and I thank God for the beauty of my being me and I don't want that anyone should want to make me someone else. We say [...] give your child the confidence to decide how to discover himself, so that's why I am in love with education. [...] because I discovered that education is all about being a learner. And when you are a learner, in the process we are all learning from each other and teaching each other."[76]

The intention of social entrepreneurs is to contribute towards making the world more humane, more liveable. The basis for their work is the good, without being do-gooders. They reflect upon what they do, are self-critical. Ravi Agarwal for instance asked: "What I do here, is this the right thing to do?"[77] The question of whether something is just is important to them:

"I am dealing with my own wanting to do something better with the world, that I want to improve the world in some way, or I want to do something better. Like I do now for the environment, but also in my own deep Self, I know, that we have to do things differently to really do that [...] we all have to change in very fundamental ways, for that to happen."[78]

Alisa del Tufo spells out the core motivation:

"[...] the most truthful way to put that is, that I believe, that people are here to be compassionate towards others and that's what I try to be and that's what I try to teach and that everything comes back to that central value."[79]

Marco Roveda and others summarise the motivation for social entrepreneurs to take action as follows: "The basis is the good, to do good."[80]

Social entrepreneurs are interested in social justice and take action to achieve it. This becomes manifest in various ways. Several remember that they always were compassionate with others, even as children. This is why some of them chose a certain field of study (e.g. economics, sociology, politics, law, education) assuming that it would help them to make changes. They reflect on social issues and develop approaches within the third sector, nationally and internationally, to try to solve them. Some of these approaches and programmes are listed below.[81]

- Courageous engagement of Founder of Ashoka (USA and worldwide), an international platform to support social entrepreneurs; www.ashoka.org – Founder: Bill Drayton.
- Prevention of violence for street children, national protection programme for children; "Financial und Social Education" for street children (in India and other nations) www.childfinanceinternational.org, www.childhelplineinternational.org, www.childline. org, www.aflatoun.org; Founder: Jeroo Billimoria.

- An eco-cultural platform including a radio, a magazine and an internet platform, to help communicate the following values, amongst others, to a wider audience: a clean environment, the realization of ideals, being happy, generosity plus information on industries which are ethical and are not only focused on making monetary profit, but also aim at supporting our wellbeing (Italy) www.lifegate.it, www.buenavistasocialgolf.org; - Founder of Scaldasole and LifeGate. Marco Roveda.
- Medical supply to villages in African countries (e.g. doctors access remote villages with boats, via the so called "floating ambulance"), provision of medical care for HIV/AIDS orphans (antiretroviral therapy) using an interdisciplinary approach; support of the Johns Hopkins Research and Rehabilitation Center in Baltimore; support of children and young adults with impaired eyesight etc (USA), www.karlkahanefoundation.org; Kahane Foundation.
- Relationship building programmes for the prevention of violence for young criminal offenders (Germany); www.violence-prevention-network.de; Founder: Judy Korn.
- Out-of-school-time education empowerment programmes for children and young adults are implemented (USA); Eco-system of new schools and nonprofits that are transforming and injecting innovation in public education; www.summeradvantage.org www.themindtrust.org; Founder of Summer Advantage (USA) Earl Martin Phalen. And children should have the same chances for success in school from the

43

start, independent of their social background. Emotional and cognitive support is provided; involving parents and paediatricians; immunization against analphabetism.He was previously CEO of Reach Out and Read; Co-Founder of BELL.

- Health support instead of administration of illness especially for those with lower income (USA); www.healthleadsusa.org; Rebecca Onie.

- Threshold activities: Using oral history and narrative to address community and social challenges. Prevention of domestic violence and child protection programmes need to work together. "Engaging the power of community" is a leitmotif to contribute towards a "more caring, just and engaged society", especially where institutional interventions fail (USA); www.connectnyc.org;   www.thresholdcollaborative.org; Founder Alisa del Tufo.

- Bank credits for the poor: Muhammad Yunus was awarded the Nobel Peace Prize for his model of microcredits which has helped millions of poor people worldwide (Bangladesh); it provides the basis for similar models in all parts of the world. Founder: www.grameenfoundation.org www.muhammadyunus.org,

- What could constructive primary school education look like? Lively, interactive classes orientated towards the things that children want to learn about, tuition focused on the environment; reform of primary schools; environmental education (India), www.parisarasha.com; Gloria de Souza.

- A forest belt around a large metropolis (Delhi, India) shall not simply be felled to satisfy the greed for profits of estate agents. The social entrepreneur took action with the result that the forest remained and now even enjoys protection. Other than that he is involved in developing solutions for the disposal of toxic waste in India; www.raviagarwal.com, www.toxicslink.org; Founder: Ravi Agarwal.

- Basic income for all; other than that engagement to show that language problems in warehouse management can be appreciated as a live model of cultural diversity (Germany and other European countries); www.unternimm-die-zukunft.de; Founder of *dm*. Götz Werner.

Other than the social initiatives and projects listed above, some of the interview partners founded additional ones, always on the intensive search for solutions to burning questions and problems. They do not accept what they consider is wrong, but campaign for justice with the aim of reaching out to as many people as possible – nationally, internationally and sometimes also globally. Their engagement for the „good" and for more justice is interwoven with the question of what gives meaning to their lives. The visions of social entrepreneurs which they managed to turn into reality demonstrate that it is not all just words. No, it is about concrete support for people in need.

They try to pass on the good which they have experienced in their lives and the help which they have received to others. Some mention that they try to spare other people the situations under which they themselves had suffered. Within this context one social entrepreneur mentioned that he will never find out why he received the help he needed.

Several social entrepreneurs remember that they always tended to be empathic towards others, even as a child. Alisa del Tufo reflects:

"[...] the sense of compassion I feel for people and any creature that needs something, has just always driven me. [...] as a child I was picking up wounded animals and taking care, that's just how I kind of have always been."

And:

"I believe that people are here to be compassionate towards others and that's what I try to be [...] and everything comes back to that central value."[82]

The social entrepreneurs find fulfillment in the fact that they are doing good. One of them agrees that he wants to continue his work as he has seen that his support makes people happy. Jeroo Billimoria has helped thousands of street children in the course of her social activities. She confirms that to do good is a vital motive for her actions and that she loves the work she does.[83]

Focusing *on the reason for action is the good* a contribution shall be noted: The psychotherapist and scientist Bernd Rieken[84] writes about the opposite of the good.[85] He reflects on the "evil" in a person and also refers to Goethe's "Faust", his view on Mephisto and Alfred Adler's observations on the drive for aggression. He talks about the everyday character of the "evil", has a historical look at the phenomenon and reviews where it might have started. Popular explanations include social injustice, the original sin or the human psyche. Looking at the function and purpose of the "evil" Goethe offers alternative explanations in his "Faust". He states that the role of Mephisto is to seduce the human being out of its inertia which it tends to be caught in. Seen in that way, Mephisto effects positive change.[86] Within this context Goetz Werner quotes Goethe, noting that the human being is in a position to distinguish the good from the evil despite Mephistopheles' art of seduction. He refers to the bet which Mephisto loses after he had wrongly believed that he could get Heinrich Faust onto his side: "And be ashamed when you have to admit: a good person in his darkness is well aware of the right path."[87]

Reason is mentioned by most of the social entrepreneurs. Goetz Werner states: „A person learns in two different ways. Via insights or via catastrophes.

[...] This has always been the way."[88] He contradicts Mephisto's argument in "Faust" that human beings are equipped with too little reason. He makes clear that sufficient human reason is available to chose the good, the "right path". This can be used accordingly by the individual and by the group.

This shows a further essential element of the success of social entrepreneurs as well as a trait of their personality: they use their mental and cognitive skills to realize constructive things. Their strong feeling for justice is supported by an inner certainty regarding what is right and what is wrong, good and not good. They feel duty bound to contribute positive things and to improve things.[89]

Most social entrepreneurs are firmly anchored in their constructive values. They realize visions supported by values based on their faith and/or humanism.

Many social entrepreneurs highlight the joy they feel doing what they do. Some have explicitly written it into the programme of their social business (see Yunus). Gloria de Souza stresses that she certainly does not sacrifice herself as many assume. Rather, her work makes her happy and fulfills her. Other social entrepreneurs argue similarly. One of them states that many people hate their jobs and that it is a blessing for him to be able to live the work he loves in the service of his personal mission[90] – the support of children's education. Critics sometimes accuse social entrepreneurs of using the good for their own purposes. However, all the interviewees are aware of the personal benefits of their activities for themselves. They do not define themselves as "do-gooders". They are called that by others. The majority are modest and tend towards understatement and thinking that they have not done enough.

Viewed psychotherapeutically, the actions of each individual are also linked to his or her subjective motivations. It has to be said that generally most business people are not primarily concerned with public welfare. It makes a large difference whether a person commits him or herself to common welfare and supports other people to overcome difficult life situations more easily or not.

For many business people, profit maximization and/or personal success is priority number one and they will pursue this aim quite radically, sometimes even when they are conscious of the fact that they are creating disadvantages for other people in doing this. A current example: numerous professions (e.g. some brokers and many others) make enormous profits to primarily satisfy their various greeds, often consciously harming others.[91]

For social entrepreneurs the purpose of their activities is to create constructive and good things for others and/or the environment (ESSE) as described in this chapter. This is a core motivation which represents a fundamental element for their success.[92]

2.4 Faith in the Human Potential for Development

Social entrepreneurs emphasise how unique humans are and are convinced that human potential can grow. In this they are positive and visionary. Judy Korn stated that one of her core motivations is her conviction that people can change.[93] Gloria de Souza felt connected to the world as a teacher. She stated that she was in love with education as, by having confidence in the children, she supported their own confidence to make decisions and to discover themselves.[94]

Ravi Agarwal speaks about the fact that the human potential for development also depends on how people live. Everybody should have the choice to decide what they want to do. But as this decision depends not only on opportunities, but also on the personality involved, the issue of the development of human potential becomes quite complicated if you think about cause and effect, he states.[95]

Earl Martin Phalen and his team of *Summer Advantage* (previously CEO of *Reach Out Read, ROR;* see also *BELL*) facilitate direct services for children (see also the *Mind Trust).* They support them in developing their potential. He feels that this is the best way to bring about social change. He worked with paediatricians who give the parents of toddlers and pre-school children suitable books, tools to read out aloud from. On the one hand this strengthens the emotional bond between the parents and their children and on the other the children are motivated to start developing an interest in education themselves. At the same time the families experience how small changes can make a huge difference for the future of the children. The children are supported in being well prepared - emotionally, knowledge-wise and socially, to enter school. This is particularly important for uneducated social groups. Earl Martin Phalen sees his personal mission in contributing towards the children feeling safe in the knowledge that they will be cared for and that they will grow up with the chance of being able to live out their potential.[96] Alisa del Tufo finds that the best way to support people in need is to move the communities into becoming the driving force behind finding the right solutions for themselves.[97]

The belief in the potential for development of an individual is deeply engrained in social entrepreneurs. They consider themselves responsible for establishing general conditions so that others can develop their individuality. Some remark that if conditions preclude this, it is inhumane and anti-social. This is why they engage in contributing things for others, hereby changing social conditions.

In their lives many social entrepreneurs experienced how family members and/or others close to them, teachers and group leaders believed in their potential and encouraged them to create their life in the best way possible. These experiences strengthened their confidence in the development potential of fellow humans.

One interview partner mentioned that she often had the feeling that she herself could be in a similarly painful life situation as those people for whom she worked. But she had the possibility to develop her potential. She therefore set herself the aim that this becomes a possibility for other people as well.

Judy Korn agrees that a firm belief in the development potential of people is vital for her work. She works on violence prevention programmes with criminal offenders.

The wish to help as many people as possible to develop their qualities is a truly heartfelt wish for most social entrepreneurs. The scientist Thomas Druyen counts the abilities of personal development, self restraint and self renewal as elements of a culture of wealth.[98] He adds that within this context there is the need for some of the elitist wealthy to change.

Everybody is unique and should be able to make his or her own decisions. Most of the interviewees feel that way. Several state that they try to expand options for others by, for instance, by strengthening the self-confidence of young people. Many social entrepreneurs consider their own life as something special, as a chance and a gift which was made possible, too, by the faith of others in their potential. It is their wish to create similar conditions for others.

A note from psychotherapeutic practice: in therapies the issue is often the development of the client's confidence in his or her various possibilities without playing down associated problems. A vital factor for the development of the client is for the therapist to maintain an optimistic-realistic attitude, even if the client himself or herself finds it difficult to keep up the hope that changes can be made. Changing attitudes, reducing suffering and supporting health[99] becomes far more successful if there is the inherent belief that the client has the potential for development.[100]

In summary, the confidence in the human potential for development is a further factor for the success of social entrepreneurs.

This chapter has described core motivations as important helpful elements for successful social entrepreneurs. They include the feeling that their work or activity has deep meaning, formative experiences which have induced them to work for good and constructive projects and, a well developed sense of justice coupled with the strong confidence in the ability of people to develop and change (ESSE).

3. Support

3.1 Honouring the Support Received

Most of the social entrepreneurs I interviewed respect and appreciate the people who have supported them. Most of them acknowledge those who have encouraged and inspired them and express this genuinely. For Muhammad Yunus, finding the cause of the debt trap of the poor was not self-evident. He is grateful that he discovered the loan sharks talking to the people in the villages.[101] Most social entrepreneurs do not see their success as based primarily on their own merits. Rather they speak of a large gift and of gratitude. "I think one of the blessings was, being able to take the lessons learned",[102] says Earl Martin Phalen. He sees that many people do a job they hate. He is grateful that he can dedicate himself professionally to his own personal mission in life.[103] Rebecca Onie and others describe their work as social entrepreneurs as a large privilege.

Social entrepreneurs do not report on their immense innovations and achievements and remain modest about their own accomplishments and the impact they have. They speak mainly about the support, sponsorship and help they have received and certainly do not take it for granted, on the contrary, they value it highly. They also thank a higher cause or life in general. They review their own course of life gratefully, the realisation of their visions and speak of gifts,[104] blessings and similar. In Earl Martin Phalen's words:

"So by or for the generosity of others namely my family, but even many others, so that's the kind of cornerstone in the work."[105]

Various studies highlight the connection between gratitude and physical well-being. The psychologist Martin Seligmann and his co-authors asked the participants of a study to write down three things every day for which they felt grateful.[106] They found that this increased the general quality of life amongst all participants. Interdependencies between the readiness to help others, gratitude and empathy were also discovered in other studies. The scientists David DeSteno and Monica Barlett had a look at the relationship between gratitude and altruism and arrived at similar conclusions.[107]

Valuing others and the positive effect this has on people's health often becomes apparent in psychotherapy.[108] Their social behaviour can be strengthened, self pity reduced and the feeling of self-worth can be increased at the same time, as action perspectives expand. People who integrate their feeling of gratitude into their value system, expand their various options to meet the challenges in their lives more constructively.

The psychologist Alex Wood and his co-authors have shown that grateful people ask others for support more readily, thus experiencing constructive coping strategies. The acknowledgement of this help leads to a positive interdependence.

One element of the success of the interview partners lies in the combination of the support they receive from their family and other people and the fact that they truly appreciate it (ESSE). Their appreciation of the help they receive supports the receipt of more help.

3.2 Actively Searching for Support

Social entrepreneurs do not hesitate to ask for support frequently in realizing their vision. This includes material support, such as funding and immaterial support, such as information. For the latter, to gain information, they often approach those affected to, seek their point of view. They also ask them for their proposals, for possible solutions to improve their situation.

They show no inhibition, neither in their private nor in their professional environment, in asking others for support or advice to be able to pursue their plans. This is particularly the case when they reach their own personal limits. Muhammad Yunus remembers how he had to knock on many doors and ask many people to get the help he needed for his project.[109] Another social entrepreneur reported how hard it was financially, especially in the start-up phase, and how he therefore turned to people he knew for help. Realising that the active cooperation of the people who are affected is essential if the support given is to be effective, Alisa del Tufo talks to them a lot to understand their point of view better. This helps her to develop better, more targeted support.

Scientists discovered that even some babies (two months and older) and small children tend to find help when they feel stressed.[110] Here the positive interdependence between the development of resilience and the ability to protest against negative stimuli becomes visible. Emmy Werner includes self protection and the ability to approach others, clearly communicating the need for support, in her description of resilience. Babies employ this ability when they cry.

Ideally by crying they receive the attention they are seeking plus an adequate reaction. According to Werner and Smith,[111] our making use of the possibilities around us represents the link between our abilities and our environment. The authors illustrate this relationship between an individual and his or her social environment with the help of a "spiral staircase model". This is an interactive model in which a child looks for the kind of environment which supports and protects it.[112] Their studies make it clear that these children start seeking attention or advice from an emotionally stable person very early on. They usually turn to people in their immediate environment, such as older siblings, grandparents, aunts, uncles, but also maybe to a favourite teacher who they see as a role model. They are very skillful in recruiting such "surrogate parents"[113] for themselves. The sociologist and systemic psychotherapist Bruno Hildebrand considers resilience as an approach which sheds more light on the strengths and abilities of people to cope with adverse conditions. He emphasises "that people and their environments do not only display injuries, but are also equipped with the strengths and abilities [...] to cope with these injuries [...]".[114] He points out that both are needed, both the strengths and the weaknesses, if we want to be able to ask for and receive support.

Most social entrepreneurs display a high degree of resilience and turn directly and immediately to others to seek help and support for the social project they are planning. They do not hesitate to ask, approaching their environment actively and repeating the process several times, if necessary. This active search for support is a feature of their success and is linked to their recognition of their personal limits (ESSE).[115]

3.3 Personal Limits and Things which Cannot be Influenced

Most social entrepreneurs are well aware of their own personal limits and of those of human beings in general. They do not overestimate themselves and remain modest despite their great successes which often have an impact on millions of people. A key element for their success is their pronounced honesty towards themselves. Ravi Agarwal states: "I am saying that it happened by circumstances outside my control." He emphasises that factors which cannot be influenced have played a role in his work as a social entrepreneur. "It just happened, I had no idea. The future takes care of itself."[116] Most social entrepreneurs treat their personal contributions towards the success of their project as relative. They state that a lot of what has happened in their lives was beyond their influence and emphasise moments which were out of their control. This attitude demonstrates a realistic assessment of circumstances and gives credit to the uncontrollable.[117]

Social entrepreneurs mention certain external developments, which were important for their path of life, but which lay well beyond their sphere of influence. These include historic events, such as the civil rights movement with Martin Luther King, the problems of integration and segregation, national and international protests of society against the Vietnam War, the anti-nuclear movement, the peace and hippie movements, Gandhi, the War of Independence and the massive famine in Bangladesh and many others. One of the social entrepreneurs concluded that it all happened the way it did, that it was not planned, it simply happened and that he had reacted to a situation. He had developed no great plan for how to approach things, but then there came this moment when he thought, yes, this could work. And it did! Social entrepreneur Ravi Agarwal illustrates this:

"I feel that some of the most important things and there are only four or five in this whole life, 50 years, have happened not because I made them happen, but because they happened. Because something around me, I am not saying it is destiny, I am saying that it happens by circumstances outside my control and then I started following the path. A simple example is [...] the forest example [...], I had no clue, if you had asked me three months before that, I am going to do this 15 years from now, I would say no way."[118]

Others tell a similar story. Bill Drayton explains that he could not have started his activities as a social entrepreneuer earlier as:

"[...] time was not right, I was not ready, the society was not ready."[119]

Gloria de Souza tells the story of a friend of hers who was a teacher in a school. When she fell ill Gloria was asked to jump in. This was the beginning of her social entrepreneur's path of reforming the school system.

In conclusion, most social entrepreneurs gain vital motivation for their work from the support of other people. They actively seek this support and honour it when it is received (ESSE). They also emphasise that some things were beyond their sphere of influence, attributing it to a higher cause or occasionally also simply to luck.

3.4 Cultural Aspects[120]

Most of the social entrepreneurs I spoke to agree that you can become active in any cultural context. Cultural differences are not significant for the success of social business. Here the cultural environment is understood both as a territorial culture and a dynamic culture, with increasingly complex economic and social systems with their respective values and meanings and the problems this brings.

Social entrepreneurs put common cultural aspects, which connect people first, before those which separate people. They quote cultural similarities, which play a role for their activities, then point to cultural differences, but return to the cultural similarities again. Most of the interview partners have made a variety of different life and professional experiences on several levels, both in the territorial, as well as the social sense and are well versed in studying cultural aspects. [121]

Poverty and people in need exist in all cultures. Cultural differences are frequently artificial and brought in from the outside. One interviewee estimates that there are 95% cultural similarities and only 5% cultural differences. Social entrepreneurs describe cultural codes as details which bring about change and create differences, but see the central values and what needs to be done as similar world-wide. Some quote territorial differences in becoming socially active. It makes a difference whether social projects are planned in Asia, South America, Africa or Northern Europe, as in some parts of the world social problems are more urgent and apparent, while in in others they are less visible. One social entrepreneur provides an example: many people consider the chances for education in Germany as sufficient. This point of view represents an obstacle for social activities in this area, as the necessity for action may seem less visible than in other countries.

Some social entrepreneurs mention the western focus on consumption, material things and self-presentation as different to that of the East, but emphasise at the same time how the West provides great support. Following the heavy earthquake in Haiti, for instance, the West gave massive emergency aid. One social entrepreneur describes different cultural attitudes. He describes the attitude in the West, as an "outcome control" attitude in contrast to the attitude in other parts of the world where people tend to think that "the future takes care of itself".[122] He experiences these differences in attitude in his professional environment when cooperation partners have different expectations.[123] These expectations are also culturally determined. In an individualistic society for instance the performance of an individual represents a higher value than in a collectivistic context.

Here and there the fact that social business is stimulated less within the societal context of a welfare state was mentioned. This, however, does not hinder people with motivation to engage themselves for public welfare anyway. As a consequence, you still come across quite a number of social entrepreneurs in Europe, too, where the social systems tend to be better developed. The necessity of a welfare state is strongly emphasised by all. At the same time some of my interview partners noted that possibly people tend to engage themselves less for others in a welfare state since part of the concept of help is delegated to State. One of the interview partners points out that, even in welfare states, some people do not receive social support. She reminds us that the state is not a person, but is composed of an assemblage of people who act or don't.[124] Another interviewee sees a similar problem in people being provided for by an unknown entity. The duty of a State is to create freedom and notes, the duty of business people is to allow freedom to develop in businesses.[125]

Several of the social entrepreneurs quote the cultural environment into which they were born as being particularly formative and stimulating. For instance the yankee culture with its traditional values and strong sense of loyalty. Being in a cultural environment which allows you to be whoever you are[126] is seen as enormously enriching. Within this context New York City and Boston, amongst other cities, are described as a "great neighbourhood", a great environment for the development of social businesses.

Additional Thoughts on the Cultural Context[127]

Ravi Agarwal whose work takes him both to Asia and to Europe is familiar with both worlds:

"Many things which we are seeing around us today are part of that cultural misunderstanding or cultural inability to understand. And I think some of these things, no matter how much we understand about our own self, very hard to break our knowledge of our history and to come to that, because we get so deeply coded into that, it is very hard to resist that yourself, even though you understand the problem. So understanding is one bit, but the inability to change your basic ways that's something much more different. I think maybe there is more attempt today than in any other time, we see more young people moving around and work in other countries and going, but I am not sure how much we really understand. I mean at a social level it's much easier. We speak similar languages [...]."[128]

He continues that in his view people travel for very material things and not for love and ethics. They want to gain something. He explains that true understanding is only possible if we really want to understand each other. This is more often than not blocked by our own wishes and expectations of others. In personal relationships we are forced to try to understand each other, as it strongly affects our own life. He describes culturally-based differences as follows:[129]

- those of a contextual, social and economic nature;
- the way we interact, communicate, work, negotiate and consider what behaviour is acceptable and what is not;
- different expectations and assumptions of different societies.

On top of that he believes that we need to face more what we have in common culturally and what separates us in a world which is becoming more and more global, as we need to find ways of living together. He assumes that all of us are experiencing a lot of change. Never before throughout human history, neither through confrontations and war, nor in times of peace has there been this degree of globalization. On a certain social level Ravi Agarwal thinks we can live together quite easily, as we speak a similar language. Also we usually share similar visions of what a good society should look and often have similar ideas, such as democracy and human rights. However, where we differ is how we move within this framework. He quotes the way we work together professionally. He states that we often do not want to acknowledge cultural differences, as a lot is judged in political dimensions. Both he himself as well as some of the other social entrepreneurs I spoke to reflected on this, finding that there is a lot of ghettoisation in this world, including in societies of wealthy countries. Earl Martin Phalen illustrates similar aspects and concludes that there seem to be more out- than in-groups.

On a deeper level Ravi Agarwal thinks we have different motivations for doing something. He mentions the idea of justice and explains that it does not necessarily have to be a spiritual one, it can also be very material.[130] The current idea that we can create justice through institutions and public bodies is a very material one. Further he states the following with regard to the cultural context:

- there are frequent misunderstandings and inabilities to understand each other;
- true understanding requires the empathic wish to want to understand the other person. This, however, is often blocked by the own wishes and expectations of the other. In personal relationships we tend to be forced to truly want to understand, as it strongly affects one's life.
- despite knowledge and awareness, it is not easy to act correctly. He sees difficulties in our breaking with our knowledge of our history and the way we are coded into it.

With these thoughts he touches upon a central question of psychotherapy, cultural sciences and adjoining disciplines: is it more the individual personal challenges or a culture-specific understanding that we are dealing with here? Emmy Werner[131] notes, that individual disposition and social backing both contribute to the resilience of a person.

The ethno-psychoanalyst Georges Devereux adopts the assumption in his interdisciplinary approach that cultural facts only become important if a person truly accepts them and considers them relevant. This relates to the relationships between individuals and the collective and the assumption that psychodynamic processes are universal, with culture-specific versions.[131a]

The interviewees all think that social entrepreneurial activities are possible in any cultural context. The concerns of social business are not dependent on cultural conditions, as they appeal to fundamental human emotions, empathy with other people and/or with the environment. Some social entrepreneurs support the inter- and transcultural aspect through their work. On the one hand they emphasise the commonalities and the humanistic factors and on the other they view cultural differences to the extent necessary, but in a constructive way.

One common factor which opposes social businesses world-wide are closed minds. And these can be found in all cultures. Everywhere.

4. Confidence - Feelings

4.1 Personal Perception and Intuition[132]

Most of the social entrepreneurs I spoke to trust their perception even if it seems to contradict external circumstances and opinions of others. They listen to their feelings closely and use them as orientation. Alisa del Tufo remembers:

"I felt like it could happen to me [...] I kind of decided then, that this would be really my life's work, that I would work in this world of helping stop violence against women and eventually against children."[133]

Gloria de Souza recalled how she knew that what she was experiencing at the moment was how teaching and schooling could actually be like. This good! Jeroo Billimoria stated: "I do, what I feel I can do."[134] And Ravi Agarwal asked: "How not to do what naturally comes to you?"[135] He continued to say:

"I think when I did engineering and business school that's where you become like a product for the world. You become very good with fitting into the economy, the work economy and that did not really excite me and felt, I did not want to spend my life doing this."[136]

Another social entrepreneur confirmed that she clearly feels and recognises what does her good and what doesn't. Earl Martin Phalen described the trust in his perception by talking about a nice experience he had. In that moment particularly and in many others, too, he said, he felt this trust and knows with every fibre of his being why he is here and that this is his meaning in life. This clarity helps him navigate through many difficult situations.

"I really feel fortunate to know to have had such clarity in terms of, so that moment and many others, those were the things that you lean on when things get hard."[137]

Most of the social entrepreneurs pointed out that at the start they didn't know whether they would be able to realise their ideas, but felt that they simply had to do something. As a consequence they went ahead, following their intuition. Alisa del Tufo remembered that she had always been an empathetic person, even as a child. She eventually became active and started to help others in need. Muhammad Yunus recalled that he did not know where this was leading to when he started the process of developing the system of microcredits:
"I didn't know how to do it, but at that moment, I thought this is the way it can be done, so I did that."[138]
He emphasised how his feeling had given him orientation and that he had simply trusted his intuition. As a consequence he was able to make extremely difficult personal decisions. He had to leave his little daughter. His wife at the time returned to her country with the child, but he did not join them, as he felt committed to staying where he was and helping the poor.

"[...] but even in that situation, I decided to stay on, I don't know why, what made me do that, but I did and I never thought, I made a mistake. I was totally convinced, I was absorbed and at that time it was not very successful, it was just the beginning."[139]

Many social entrepreneurs distance themselves from the expectation of others and trust their own perception. Bill Drayton remembered negotiations with representatives of a tobacco company in his previous position as a manager and how they had tried to influence the negotiations. So trusting his intuition and having had prepared himself thoroughly he had the courage to confront them and uncover their unfair practices: "This sounded all wrong to me."[140]

Ravi Agarwal described his feelings when the enormous forest belt surrounding Delhi was under threat to be destroyed to pave the way for real estate developers: "I felt this was wrong."[141] He listened to his feeling and decided to act accordingly, with success. Most social entrepreneurs use their inner values and their feeling of whether something seems wrong as orientation. Some explicitly mention that they trust their intuition.

This is an important pillar of support for fundamental issues in their lives. One of my interview partners summarised the attitude of most social entrepreneurs towards their work as follows: "How not to do what naturally comes to you?"[142]

Angelantonio Ferrandina, existential, spiritual- and life counsellor, pointed out the importance of intuition and its resources.[143] He emphasises that more attention needs to be given to these resources in therapeutic practice as well as in research and education.

The pychotherapist Alfried Längle,[144] too, highlights the intuitive sensibility with which people are equipped, telling us what makes sense and what doesn't. Children for instance are usually reluctant to do something which they consider senseless. A healthy environment will support this sensibility of theirs. A child's sensibility also comes to light when adults are cynical. Children do not understand cynicism, an attitude which is usually adopted when we have lost trust in our own feelings. For children this feels strange.

Werner and Smith and other scientists have shown that people who have been born into difficult family situations or problematic environments can develop strong trust in their personal perception, too. If sciences paid more attention to the results of research on resilience, some persistent popular theories which try to reduce who we are to the importance of the first years of our life would become unsustainable (see also research results of Jens Asendorpf).[145]

Most of the social entrepreneurs speak about "not-knowing". This is where their sub-conscious knowledge comes into play. A certain knowledge is there, is perceived intuitively and is proven by their actions. In some situations intuition can be seen as subconscious knowledge. There are certain areas in our life which are beyond our control.[146] One of the social entrepreneurs stated that he wanted to experiment and give his life a chance. This means that he listens closely to the ideas as they crop up.

He said it makes him feel modest to be able to trust. He considers it a privilege. What he means is that so many people are trapped in their problems and life situations that they do not use this ability.

Thomas Druyen defines "wealth" multi-dimensionally:

"The fascinating thing about the concept of wealth is that it refers to external splendour on the one hand, but also allows insight into one's own soul. Wealth in this sense is not only what we own, but always who we are, too. It is not only about property and possessions, but also about talents, life planning and the ability to set priorities. If we talk about a culture of wealth within this context, we need to include all values which we consider essential for a life of fulfillment ... Our wealth is our mind, our will and our feelings. If we use them in organizing our life we increase our power of managing our own existence."[147]

In conclusion most social entrepreneurs place large value on their personal perception, their feelings and their intuition in all their projects and can thus certainly be considered "wealthy".

4.2 Being Touched

The interview partners spoke about deep emotions, inner turmoil, anger, desperation and shock in the face of injustice. But they also spoke about the great joy they felt when they saw how they had managed to make someone happy with what they were doing. In Muhammad Yunus's words: "So I did that and it made them very happy and I wanted to continue this."[148] So he carried on and developed the model of microcredits, jointly with others, and now supports social business throughout the world. He described his original feeling of shock and desperation and how it stirred him up inside when he saw how ignorant the bank managers were towards the poor. He confronted them and decided to take action:

"I am very agitated, how can you leave them to the loan-sharks, this is your organization which is supposed to lend money and you say that cannot be done. You don't even try. So I started agitating against them, I went to all the people in the bank to knock at their doors, [...]."[149]

Ravi Agarwal described how a plan to undertake massive environmental destruction made him so angry that he felt that he simply had to do something about it.

"Firstly I was very angry, it made me really angry that somebody can destroy the forest. [...] I don't know why I was so angry [...] I have this deep relationship with nature, the idea of nature and it agitates me inside. [...] somebody is doing something which I think this is unjust, unfair, I get agitated inside. I feel this is not right. And then I need to do something about it."[150]

Alisa del Tufo remembered her consternation, too:

"I was very upset by the fact that as a domestic violence organization we weren't really thinking very much about the children and I was very upset that here was a woman who had been beaten for so long and she'd never been in one of the domestic violence programs."[151]

One of the interviewees described the pain that he had experienced in a key situation and decided: "I didn't want other people to feel the way I felt in that moment."[152]

Another was highly frustrated with his former work as an entrepreneur in the profitable IT business. He remembers his emotions at the time and how churned up he was. He had the feeling that there was no way he could stay in that job and that he had to quit this type of profession.[153]

Others spoke about the anger or shock they felt in the face of certain events, but also about their feelings of happiness triggered by things that had happened. Almost all interviewees described intense and deeply emotional experiences – negative as well as positive ones – which motivated them to continue their work, to carry on. Feelings were particularly intense if certain events or experiences contradicted or completely agreed with their inner values.

Emotions such as anger and grief and also positive emotions such as joy and happiness are catalysts for social entrepreneurs to get active and tackle even difficult situations. Their actions are driven by their values. Inner or external conflicts and strong emotions can have a particularly long-lasting effect and influence future decisions.

Everybody has tough experiences in his or her life and goes through crises. What all of the interview partners have in common is strong resilience. They have all confronted difficult phases in their lives or catastrophic events, such as violence, hunger or environmental destruction with an unusual portion of courage. The psychotherapist Rosemarie Welter-Enderlin views resilience from a therapeutic perspective. For her, being human means occasionally standing on the edge of an abyss.[154] The researcher Froma Walsh identified a connection between crises and difficulties and a resulting boost of moral awareness, the development of new aims in life and engagement and support for people in difficult situations.[155]

The work of most of the social entrepreneurs was highly inspired by being touched very deeply by experiencing true joy through certain events, but also injustice and suffering. In conclusion, intense life experiences were an effective motivation for them, especially if these experiences touched upon their fundamental values (ESSE).

4.3 Spiritual Dimension

For most of the interview partners the spiritual dimension is an important part of their way of life and professional engagement. The individual approaches towards spirituality vary. For some it gives meaning to their life.

Several of the social entrepreneurs feel that if we ignore our spiritual dimension, we reduce our being human. Muhammad Yunus states:

"Human beings are not machines. Human beings are multidimensional, so among all those dimensions there maybe a spirituality [...] it is part of human being, reflect who I am, why am I here, what do I do."[156]

One of his books contains a chapter with the title "God is in the Details". In this chapter he describes his cooperation with the company Danone to produce nutrient-rich yoghurt for the poor. He disagrees with the idea, which is propagated by certain theories, that we only have a physical dimension. For him, this is a limited view of humans.

"The moment you open up you'll see so many varieties of actions coming in, it is a selfless business, a social business, so that's the point I was making, that selflessness is built into human being."[157]

Some social entrepreneurs speak about how spirituality in general is part of their life. Others explicitly mention their religious affiliation (for instance Hinduism, Islam or Christianity). Alisa del Tufo recounted how she first studied Buddhism, reflecting on social justice and her own role in the world and finally decided to continue with studies leaning towards Christianity:

"I was more interested in how peoples values or their faith affected how they live their life, how they solve their problems, how they dealt with life's difficulties. So I ended up going to a Christian seminary.[158]

The social entrepreneurs emphasise what is common to religions. They underline those aspects which connect religions and speak about the positive values of spirituality. Gloria de Souza sees her work as a social entrepreneur anchored in Christian values. The education institution which she founded is orientated towards Christianity and uses an "interfaith" approach, working with both fundamental Muslims and Hindus without being missionary. The aim is to increase awareness and prevent any form of extremism. Both Muslims and Hindus cherish the high quality of the Christian educational opportunities which they need for their own schools. She illustrates:

"In the process we are able to say, see, what you believe for the goodness of your religion is wonderful, but use your influence also to see, that jihad for instance should not be something that is promoted. Holy wars, whether they are Christian, Muslim or Hindu holy wars, whatever, can this be something that is really bringing harmony and peace? And if it is not bringing harmony and peace, how can we see that side of the religion that's something that we got to promote?"

And adds:

"I personally feel that I don't have to convert people. That for me being Christian doesn't mean that I have to tell a Muslim, you should convert to Christianity or a Hindu, you should convert to Christianity, No. For me what it means to be Christian is to live this all embracing loving, caring way of being one community before God. I feel that when religions divide, that is wrong, that is harmful, so people sense that. They feel, this is an organization which is secular, they have no religious label. However we noted Christian principals will provide that, but also

Christian principles that we love and it is them that are making it possible for us to work together."[159]

Jeroo Billimoria who was socialized in a Hindu context summarizes: "I believe a lot in God and spirituality. I think everything you do is guided by God."[160] In 2011 Bill Drayton held a public talk on the topic of social entrepreneurs in the Radiokulturhaus in Vienna, Austria. When the moderator asked him whether his concept is backed by a rational or a spiritual idea he replied: "It's both, I don't know how you could divide them."[161]

The interviewees think about who they are, why they are here and what they are doing. These thoughts are reflected in their work. Earl Martin Phalen emphasises that his spiritual basis supports his work:

"I mean, if you believe that we are all God's creatures then you can't rationalize the way we treat one another. My spiritual and faith basis are cornerstones to the work that I do."[162]

And in Götz Werner's words:

"These human existential questions 'Where do I come from? Where am I going to?' These are the basic questions after all. How am I to lead my life in a meaningful way if I don't ask myself these questions? If we think that there is a black hole in front of us and a black hole behind us we will never get anywhere. We will remain absolute materialists. [...] We have to acknowledge the reality of the spiritual."[163]

Gloria de Souza describes the influence of spirituality on her life:

"The Christian way of life is what drives me. What is the Christian way of life? For me it is not the rituals, but it is just this idea of love one another and be there for each other and find your own self and the commitment to oneself. But in the process are you also giving to others what you have taken from nature and society and from people [...]. That has inspired me. The Atma, the soul and for me the soul is nothing but the presence of God within oneself. If we are conscious of that, whether we call it God or whatever else. Some of my dearest friends are agnostics, they say they don't believe in God, but I know when I see their lives so full of truth and beauty and goodness and wisdom, though they may not go to a temple or a church or anything like that, but for them, the acknowledgement of truth and duty and goodness and wisdom is the acknowledgement of the source of all that, whatever we want to call it. [...] So regardless of religion, you will see that there are some Hindus, some Muslims, some Christians."[164]

Ravi Agarwal who was socialised in the Hindu context explains:

"I was grown in a family with deep spiritual values. Not necessarily religious values, but deep spiritual values. And spiritual values drive me more than material values, even today material values do not really drive me. I think they are necessary, but then I will not sacrifice my life for them. - Deep down I believe in this idea of spiritual Self, that my material existence is only part of my whole existence, not the only existence. And there are many more other forces or vibrations around me and I am very keen to know what they are. And I am very keen to know what's the boundary, who am I in the whole thing."

He continues:

"I have been in a church, I have been in a mosque, I have been in a Sikh temple, I don't feel any difference. It's really for me spirituality, is about energy and about energy bigger than me, so if I wanna put it very simply, it's about that I am smaller than something else. […] This is my spiritual idea of the selfs and that could have many forms. I am more interested in the core idea of the need for religion and religion itself, not about the culture and the culture of various religious codes and practices [...] because we identify so closely with religion, many people do, and I think it's an evolutionary question I think, that means not engaging with the real idea, but are doing exactly what religion is telling you not to do."[165]

Some social entrepreneurs describe themselves as not spiritual. The pillar for their work is humanism and the values which were passed on to them by their families of origin. One shares the same values as her christian partner, including being respectful towards each other and nurturing the relationship. Another one mentions similar aspects. She feels a close connection to the Jewish, but not in a religious sense.

Most of the social entrepreneurs desire an active relationship with something higher, with God or however you want to call it, plus constructive relationships with their fellow human beings. Some of them regret that many people pretend to act in the name of a religion, but actually do the precise opposite of what religion would want them to do.[166] One social entrepreneur added that people love to create a large spectrum of new gods. Some turn science into their religion.

This chapter speaks about the spiritual which expressly does not mean the esoteric. This needs to be emphasised, as in everyday language both terms are often mixed up.[167] What most interviewees have in common is that the values connected to faith, which are integrated into their lives, are much more important to them than the rituals of the respective religions. They describe the importance of the spiritual dimension in their lives in very similar words, despite their different religious affiliations and cultural backgrounds. One thing is noticeable though: Asian interview partners and some from the US talk about spirituality more openly than the European ones. It should also be noted that none of them works for a denominational organisation.

In his essay "Meaning: From a Live of Inner Consent to the Detection of Spirituality", the existential analyst and logotherapist Alfried Längle[168] discusses the importance of spirituality for a fulfilled life. One of the biggest questions of every human being is: "Why am I here?" He thinks that our wish to try to understand the "why" and the sense and meaning is entrenched in our mental potential and spiritual dimension. Following Viktor

Frankl, Längle reflected on this non-physical force in combination with our freedom and called this a further "spiritual capacity".

The psychologist Froma Walsh identified transcendency and spirituality as a source of resilience.[169] Other experts including Imber-Black, Roberts, Whiting, or Werner and Smith came to similar conclusions. They discovered that mental resources embedded in spirituality and meditation plus our feeling of togetherness are sources of resilience factors.[170]

The majority of the interviewees draw motivation, meaning in what they do and perseverance from a spiritual dimension. They obtain power and orientation from being embedded in it.[171] They feel part of a whole and perceive something greater beyond their own self. Walsh mentions that many live out their spiritual resources in a personal connection with something bigger, including nature, music and art and do not depend on a certain church affiliation. Several social entrepreneurs have noticed a societal change. A move from a compulsory material culture towards one which is more spiritual. We are moving towards a lifestyle with other values.

Most social entrepreneurs see spirituality as part of humans. They clearly see their work as serving a higher entity. Their personal engagement in their work stems from inner values derived from their spiritual beliefs and values (ESSE). These values are a source of inspiration for them.

4.4 Compassion

Social entrepreneurs are interested in other people. For the interviewees human compassion and empathy is a central concern. Alisa del Tufo recognises the central value of people being compassionate towards each other:

"[...] the most truthful way to put it is, that I believe, that people are here to be compassionate towards others and that's what I try to be and that's what I try to teach and that everything comes back to that central value." – "So I started talking to the women that were coming to the sanctuary about their experiences being a mother. How being a mother affected their decisions to stay or their decisions to leave, whether it made it easier or harder or whatever. I wanted to understand this much more deeply."

Social entrepreneurs really want to understand and find the root of problems. Speaking to the people they are committed to help is essential. Alisa del Tufo, for instance, sought the opinion of many women faced with violence.

"So I interviewed 45 women who were mothers and were abused - to more deeply understand the staying for the children, leaving for the children, how their children impacted all these decisions for them. There was so much information that they gave me. I learned a lot of what they thought about the overlapping issues, but I also learned that only two of them had ever called a battered women shelter. This was in 1991. So two lightbulbs went on. One was that there was enormous opportunity to educate people about the overlap and there was enormous opportunity to help women understand how the violence was impacting their children. That was one set of insights. The other was that there were all these women and children out there, who were experiencing violence, who were not using the services. So we had to find new and different ways of reaching them."[172]

So she learns from them and improves the services she provides by the new insights she has gained. Social entrepreneurs make use of new findings from conversations with persons concerned and develop new ways to provide a more targeted support. They are good and active listeners and very willing to learn. They listen to be able to provide better help. Judy Korn described the following:

"I kept on coming across young men who questioned my role as a woman and who did not want to have any dealings with me as they didn't consider me an equal partner. This was a clash in conceptions of values. But finally I did manage to access them through my personal interest in building a relationship with them."[173]

Social entrepreneurs are interested in the causes of problems. Most of them, though, are not only excellent listeners, but express their own feelings, too, are compassionate and make people feel that, just by the way they are. They leave the role of the expert and ask the people concerned what they need and what they want. This is how they get to the bottom of difficulties and learn from the people for whom they engage themselves. They do not place themselves "above" the person who is currently in need.

Social entrepreneurs usually communicate openly with the people they are trying to support but also with other people within the system they work in. The ability to express oneself is described as part of resilience by Froma Walsh.[174] Social entrepreneurs share their own feelings. On the emotional level this creates authentic compassion which connects people. On the other hand if a helper expresses pity for the other person, she or he has classified this person as helpless. This evokes defense, as the person concerned is reluctant to accept the role of a victim, since it gives rise to the feeling of being powerless. Contrary to this, compassion and true empathy make the other feel understood and implies that she or he is not alone. This in itself makes a remarkable positive difference for people in difficult situations. Authentic communication as described is particularly important in psychotherapy, too, for the same reasons. Unfortunately sometimes too little attention is paid to this. For instance if a person remains stuck in his or her role as a victim, this will hinder lasting change. Often somebody affected finds it hard to leave this role, as she or he has integrated an apparent subjective benefit of the suffering into this sort of behavioural pattern.

Many social entrepreneurs receive ideas and approaches to solutions from those asking for help. This allows a direct and concrete focus on the causes of the problems and what can be done about them. One social worker for instance found a solution to a central problem after having talked to a child.

Bill Drayton spoke about the many dialogues he had with the social entrepreneurs of the global platform

Ashoka which he founded. He underlined one particularly characteristic trait of many of them – that they listen and ask questions.

"They are equally focused on 'How-to-Questions'. Their path is one of constant, either if it is listening and adjusting, creating, problem solving and listening again. They are very very good listeners as a result."[175]

I noticed the same with the social entrepreneurs I spoke to. They ask questions, listen intently to the answers and learn from others. In a certain sense they do not see themselves as the experts, but those for whom they work.

Most of the social entrepreneurs combine authentic compassion with active listening. (ESSE) These acquired and deeply engrained qualities are one of their main characteristics.

4.5 Unconscious Factors

Unconscious factors can play a part in social business, too.[176] It is important to note that the aspects outlined below are not seen as isolated elements, but rather as a possible part of the whole picture. Here and there additional material from public talks or publications of some of the social entrepreneurs has been consulted.

Success is Socialised

Social entrepreneurs are particularly aware of the community and the environment. With regard to the success of their activities, they place themselves and their actions which have contributed to this success into the background. They usually use the word "we". They mostly say "it could be" and "possibly", although they are equipped with above average competencies – both human and related to the subject matter. This behaviour shows a certain modesty. Successes are presented as joint achievements. This might not come as a surprise for people socialized in a collectivist cultural environment. However, a similar trait is also seen in social entrepreneurs from the individualistic US context. Professor Muhammad Yunus's comment to the enormous global recognition of him and his work is that he is simply a symbol for social business. He emphasises the collaboration of many and the common vision which achieved this success.

Most of the social entrepreneurs I interviewed socialize their successes, but personalize failure. The mental dynamic behind this and this inner attitude can be considered a further element for their success (ESSE). Many people behave completely the other way around.

Deep Trust in Perception and Intuition

From a psychotherapeutic point of view, the trust of some of the social entrepreneurs in their inner perception is deeper than they express in words. Several of them mentioned that they often don't know why they behaved in this or that way. Some say that their work gives them energy.

"I do it, because that's the way it comes to me and that's what gives me life and that's what gives me energy, but I don't really understand it why I am doing it."[177]

Although they sometimes state that they "do not know", for instance with regard to "how it shall go on", an inner certainty can be felt. This can be interpreted as implicit knowledge. They trust their perception, are courageous and feel that they want to do something, can do something: "I do what I feel I can do."

Part of the strong self-confidence of the interview partners can be traced back to their deep trust (ESSE), which gives them inner support, especially in precarious situations.

Expectations

Some of the interview partners touched upon the expectations of individual family members, articulated or not, which they tried to meet. In some cases the wish to be acknowledged by a certain person can play a role for social engagement. Most people have the desire to be acknowledged. This can be coupled with high ethical personal standards. Concrete expectations of important people in one's life often remain unspoken and/or expectations are sometimes only imagined and do not actually exist. But even these imagined expectations can be just as constructive and motivating. One of the social entrepreneurs describes an implicit motto of his family of origin: "better be the best" and emphasises that nobody in his family ever demanded that of him.[178]

Rebecca Onie considers it a great privilege to be a social entrepreneur. As a child she was inspired by the role model of her father. After an event, where he had been invited as a speaker, he encouraged her by saying: "One day this could be you."[179]

Of course social entrepreneurs also manage to distance themselves from the expectations of others in many ways. This may seem paradoxical in the face of what has been said before. However, the ability to distance themselves usually does not refer to an important person in their lives, but to their wider environment.

Feelings of Guilt

Sometimes feelings of guilt can be part of the motivation for activities. Social entrepreneurs quote the support they have received from others which is why they are doing so well. One of the interview partners explained that through social engagement the unsettling feeling of being fortunate, whilst so many others are not, becomes more remote. For some this sense of being fortunate might evoke feelings of guilt and reinforce the desire to do something for others. On the other hand a subjectively perceived personal disadvantage can be compensated with mental and social strengths, using it as a resource.

Several of the interview partners started to help others early on, as they were growing up. Social entrepreneurs feel co-responsible for others. This sense of responsibility goes very deep: "I would give my life [...]"[180] one social entrepreneur said in describing his attitude, meaning the children whom he is helping. Their commitment with which they support others is without compromise. Some said that they felt that their actions help to make others happy. For some this was one incentive to continue. In others it might be some connection to open questions surrounding their own lives. Another motivation is their contribution to more social justice through intensive social engagement. One of the personalities said that she felt that she could be hit by the same fate which had affected those in need of help:

"I felt like it could happen to me [...] I kind of, decided then, that this would be really my life's work, that I would work in this world of helping stop violence against women and eventually against children".[181]

Some social entrepreneurs are completely aware of the factors mentioned here. In some the depth of trust in their inner perception and the resulting consequence of their actions might actually be stronger than they are fully aware of or actually expressed. In conclusion, a few unconscious factors may provide additional motivation for the activities of social entrepreneurs.

5. Decisions

5.1 Personal Responsibility and Willingness to Take Risks

Many people want change, but de facto do little to achieve it. In contrast, social entrepreneurs actively try to turn their ideas and visions into reality. In their lives they often make uncomfortable decisions. They are willing to take risks and adhere to their values in what they do, even in precarious situations, without knowing the consequences of their decisions. They are guided by insights. They use crises in their lives for personal development, for instance to become more resilient. Sometimes these crises involve very painful experiences, such as separations, violence, illness, death and other deep events. One of the "change agents" can be death, as, faced with death, everything else falls into perspective. Social entrepreneurs extract important insights from difficult life situations. They commit themselves to their plan, against all odds, seeing it as their mission and responsibility. Some refuse well-paid job offers, often material comforts have no priority for them. They act authentically, according to their values. They are not willing to make compromises, even if their decisions have adverse consequences. They jump into action without being able to rely on a "safety net" which is usually unavailable at the time. Devaluing comments from others about themselves or their plans do not deter them from following their vision.

Social entrepreneurs drop certain activities if these

contradict their social or ecological concerns. They dedicate time and energy to their vision without compromise. These visions include e.g. obtaining credits for the poor, so that they can escape the poverty trap, arranging for chances for the education of children from underprivileged families, resocialising juvenile delinquents, setting up child protection programmes and prevention of violence programmes and effecting environmental protection.

Their inner values guide their whole life, including their decisions for social engagement, and shield them from opportunism. They do not allow negative external conditions to hinder them to continue, they also gain own personal growth out of difficult situations and increase their competency in dealing with professional crises.

Werner und Smith examined the relationship between individual protective factors and their environment and found that resilient women and men act self responsibly and react actively to adverse circumstances. They actively look for people and possibilities to overcome a difficult situation.[182] Experiences from psychotherapeutic practice illustrate similar phenomena. People who leave their roles as victims manage to change destructive behavioural patterns more easily and more frequently, thus managing to reduce their own suffering.[183] The role of the victim implies powerlessness and it increases suffering as the affected person remains blind to her or his opportunities and other options. Only when that person leaves the role of the victim and starts to actively look for possibilities around her or himself do perspectives open up as well as ways out. This strengthens self-confidence and optimism. These experiences of self-efficacy increase the competency of the individual and open up additional possibilities.

Social entrepreneurs display a particularly high degree of personal responsibility. This quality marks their entire biography and it is something they often speak about. On top of that they are self critical, often scrupulously honest towards themselves and do not succumb to self pity, even in difficult situations. They don't care about losing face or status and even take job losses into account. Social entrepreneurs consider their own integrity a priority, especially when discrepancies arise between their professional tasks and their values. They are authentic. One of the social entrepreneurs I interviewed described his emotional state while he was a successful businessman as deadly. He realized that this was due to the priority of the company to make money. Deciding that he could not endure this unsatisfying situation any longer, he changed his life. He started to put his energy into environmental protection and started up a social business for toxic waste disposal in an Asian metropolis. He described his ability to take on personal responsibility as consoling.

Research on resilience shows that the active attitude towards problems has a substantial influence on resilient people. Social entrepreneurs face challenges actively. At the same time they manage to distance themselves from the judgment of others, both within their private and professional environment. They ignore devaluing comments such as: "You are mad, stupid, naïve, self-exploiting, etc." For them the responsibility towards those they feel committed to has priority.

As I mentioned previously, most people tend to personalise success, but socialise failure. This is quite a widespread societal behaviour. This means if something goes wrong, the others are fault, however, if something is a success it is claimed as a personal success. I am sure that all of us have experienced this. It starts with simple things between one person and another, continues in the professional environment and then, on a grand scale, it also happens nationally and globally.

Sometimes people including decision-makers in organisations, corporations, financial institutions, provinces and States like to shove the blame for mistakes and failure onto others. Put bluntly, taking responsibility for misconduct and remaining liable for the damage caused is not *en vogue*.[184]

The social entrepreneurs that were interviewed usually behave the other way around. If something did not work or if mistakes occurred they look for the cause in themselves mainly and try to change or do something to remedy the situation. In the rare instances that they do utter critique it is usually in general terms and is sometimes coupled with astonishment over how other people behave. For instance Marco Roveda stated that he thinks it is strange that many demand things of others and of companies which they themselves are not willing to deliver.[185] For social entrepreneurs, personal responsibility implies a certain co-responsibility for people in need, a contribution to improve their situation. They feel obliged to become active and do not simply accept it if mistakes in the system cause more people to suffer.

Many social entrepreneurs are truly willing to take a risk and are particularly conscientious. Their deep feeling of professional responsibility in what they do is connected with their set of values. Both those who are socialized in a collectivist context, as well as those socialized in a more individualistically orientated environment have a remarkable sense of responsibility.

Successful social entrepreneurs are capable of self-reflection and self-critique which is apparent in their strong sense of responsibility (ESSE). This requires the readiness to realise one's own mistakes and to deal with the consequences in a constructive way.

5.2 Realists

Social entrepreneurs rigorously face realities and do not shy away from them in pursuing their vision. They earnestly seek answers to problematic situations on all different levels. This attitude is also apparent in their practical and unconventional methods for finding solutions to the tasks at hand. They do not allow illusions to delude them and, remain idealistic with regard to their visions. Goetz Werner describes illusion as an adversary power which makes us believe that we are safe. To illustrate his point he uses a metaphor from the world of boxing. "Every boxer knows that he must never stand firmly on both two feet, otherwise he will fall over as soon as he is touched." He continues to say:

"We have to find the middle. We can only live in the middle between the poles of the past and the future. The nostalgics are stuck in the past and the euphorics lift off, painting the future in colours which are too brilliant [...]. And what both of them miss is the presence, the here and now."

"The nostalgics always speak of the past and use killer phrases such as: 'What do you mean, we have been doing this for the past 10 years.' Or: 'That has never worked before.' Within companies you hear statements like these all day. The euphoric exclaims: 'We have to do this and this and this and this, too...' Both miss out on the presence, but we can only get active and do something in the presence."[186]

This is a human problem which is a common issue in psychotherapy. Many people are affected by it. Clinging on to the past opposes change and prevents personal development. To live in the "here and now" means to accept that change is an important constant factor of life. Sometimes this can be hard.

An increased sense of reality and being in the "here and now" is only possible if we let go of the past, of things that burden us and hold us back. According to Walsh,[187] resilience also consists of realising what can be done, what is possible and feasible and on the other hand what cannot be changed. I think in particular, accepting it makes a big difference. A person with hope consciously confronts reality. This activates energy and power to reduce risks and increase the chances for success.

Social entrepreneurs are very realistic. This is manifested in their concrete and real social projects. This is how they find wide-ranging solutions to social problems and environmental concerns. Their unsparing realism helps them to overcome obstacles and develop farsightedness (ESSE). This is a further element of their success.

5.3 Out of the Box Thinking

Social entrepreneurs look for ways to turn their visions into reality. They are creative and do not remain stuck in traditional ways and patterns of thinking. Their creativity is stimulated particularly when traditional approaches fail or are in conflict with their values. They break out of the usual behavioural norms and look for better alternatives. They don't remain within the boundaries of what is known, but enter unknown territories where they literally think *"out of the box"*. One social entrepreneur describes this attitude as a core principle of his without which he would not be able to evolve and be creative.[188]

For most of the interviewees their creativity developed when they were faced with limits. This may sound paradoxical, but here is an example to illustrate this: Muhammad Yunus described how he generally developed unusual ideas after having tried all other possibilities and failed. Searching for a way for the poor to receive credits he realized that he could not rely on the traditional bank system to help him. During a lecture he delivered at the Academy of Sciences in Vienna in 2009, he was asked how he had developed his creative idea of the microcredits. His short and clear answer was: "Out of sheer desperation."[189]

He discovered how the poor remain caught in a vicious circle of debts, as they are not classified as creditworthy by established banks and are therefore forced to turn to loan sharks. After many unsuccessful attempts to try and find a solution for this dilemma within the traditional banking system he started to think and act beyond the limitations of usual bank practices. He described how his ideas started to develop: "After I took the first step, the second followed and with it an idea of the third step."

Earl Martin Phalen asks the visionary question why it should not be possible to establish a global standard for children's education, when it is possible to establish a global standard for hotel chains.[190] Most of the personalities I interviewed think beyond the usual framework and concepts, particularly in critical situations and emergencies.

Social entrepreneurs operate unconventionally and display unusual ways of thinking and behaving (ESSE). In their social businesses this creativity is commonplace. This exceptional flexibility clearly sets them apart from most people and institutions which frequently hinder them in realizing their entrepreneurial visions.

Social entrepreneurs do not allow themselves to be deterred from their plans by others, even if they keep on being told that their plan is impossible.

They try many different possibilities to solve a particular problem. They take small steps which eventually lead them to their goal. They do not give up albeit they may be faced with hostility and the repeated message that their plan is not doable. They do not cease to look for ways to realize their visions.

Gloria de Souza recognized the power and efficiency of an education model which was presented at a seminar she attended. This model focused on environmental issues and had a practical orientation. Despite much resistance she managed to convince her colleagues to implement it jointly. This is how she brought about some reforms of part of the school system in India.

Social entrepreneurs are very clear in what they do, despite others criticizing them and trying to hold them back. Earl Martin Phalen stated: "I know that people think that is not possible."[191] Others report of their experiences of hearing again and again that the plan won't work. Still they continue, undeterred. This implies a strong will and perserverance despite pessimistic statements by others, discouraging facts and adverse conditions. This perseverance and the courage to continue even though conditions are unfavourable and then emerging from the experience double strong is an ability of resilient people. Resilience does not simply consist of a positive feeling, but of the ability to face the difficulties in life and grow in the process.[192]

In another case a social entrepreneur had to make a particularly hard decision either to stay with his partner and child or to fight for the many poor, his deep social concern. He decided to continue his fight for the poor, although his activities had not yet lead to success. Years later a close relationship developed between father and daughter. She understood his former decision and is now active as a social entrepreneur and artist herself and supports her father.[193] At the time when he made his decision this could not have been foreseen.

Many social entrepreneurs are courageous, take action and invest everything despite being rejected by others. They have little time for sceptics and pay no attention to opinions of others who try to dissuade them from their plans. They do not let their feeling of self-worth depend on the recognition by others. For this a deep conviction that their social endeavours are literally essential is required. Tirelessly they look for ways to implement their plans. These factors and their central motivations based on their values give them the necessary energy to persevere (ESSE).

In the preceding paragraphs of this chapter mainly the entrepreneurial abilities of social entrepreneurs have become apparent. It comes as no surprise that they include classic entrepreneurial characteristics such as the willingness to take risks, the ability to take decisions, a healthy portion of realism, creativity and stamina (ESSE).

6. Obstacles – Difficulties

Social entrepreneurs speak of the endless difficulties and phases of frustration and anger in the course of pursuing their visions. Despite this, they continue on their mission. Bill Drayton said about social entrepreneurs: "They will only be satisfied, if they have changed the system across their society or across society in general."[194]

In Asia and the US "problems" are frequently referred to as "challenges". Some say that they are continuously confronted with contradictions and difficulties, with forces which try to dissuade them from what they are doing. In the social entrepreneurial reality there are tons of difficulties which have to be overcome. So what is the motivation to continue their social engagement with such intensity? Earl Martin Phalen states: "Our work is so challenging, that you don't persevere, unless you have really deep roots in terms of *why* you are doing it."[195]

The most common obstacles for the realization of visions of social entrepreneurs are:
– mentalities
– lack of confidence
– time
– financial issues
– corruption

6.1 Mentalities

Social entrepreneurs see people's mentalities as the biggest problem. Convincing people of the idea is always a big issue. In the interviews with them they illustrated this point with many different examples. For instance institutions and authorities are based on certain mentalities. People are trained to think the way they are used to, the way they have always thought. One of the interview partners spoke of people freezing their minds. Others used similar metaphors. Education and school systems are founded on this way of thinking.

Some reported that people don't believe that their projects are at all possible. Each one of my interview partners has frequently heard the comment "that won't work". Goetz Werner said: "At the beginning I was told: 'that won't work.' My answer was: 'You will see that it will.' "[196]

Through her work, Gloria de Souza tried to change ways of thinking. She considered what she had achieved as a mere drop in the ocean compared to what still needs to be done (referring to reforming the school system in India). Muhammad Yunus summarises:

"I would say the biggest problem over years that I see, if I have to sum up with one word, it will be the mindset. The people as they grow up, they make their mindset solid, so they interpret everything in terms of what they have been trained to think."

and:

"[...] mindset as one word and the institutions built on the basis of that mindset. Very difficult. It is very difficult

> to change the ideas behind the institutions like banks, businesses and so on, because they are traditionally doing the things that they did. They have been trained to do exactly what others before them had done."[197]

He remains optimistic. Now, with the help of the new technologies we can experience different parallel realities in real time. This increases our mental flexibility, he thinks. In the past, information was passed on to many people by one single person. Today we have a direct exchange and stronger and closer confrontation with other ways of thinking.

Social entrepreneurs see a large obstacle in trying to convince people as mindsets are frozen and rules and regulations are interpreted unduly restrictively. They quote the judicial system as an example where officers frequently interpret the legal scope of discretion very narrowly. The unwilling often use rules and regulations as a pretext to hinder positive changes in the system. As a consequence, nonsensical processes are maintained so that the automatisms people are used to can be continued unimpeded. Institutions need to keep busy, as their employees cannot be sacked. Measures which were sensible originally, such as the protection against dismissal, seem contra productive now, as they make change more difficult. The majority of social entrepreneurs share the opinion that people tend to be sceptical towards change. Many prefer to stay with what they're used to.

Goetz Werner describes his experiences as follows:

"Good ideas don't fail because they're not good. They fail because people are not open to them. The human way of thinking, our way of thinking is so set, so frozen that we are often trapped in a prison of imagination. Many people are like that, that's the problem and [...] this is actually unchristian. Change, evolution is Christian [...]."[198]

Many social entrepreneurs consider dominant world views as materialistic and based on a set way of thinking. Inflexible. They see people's mindsets as the biggest obstacles they are faced with in pursuing their social entrepreneurial activities.

Most have made the experience that it is hard to realize new ideas. Many people dismiss great, new ideas and are closed to them, as they are boxed in by their thinking habits and comfortable traditions. The solutions to social problems require a change of awareness. Goetz Werner believes: "To run a business means running awareness."[199] He explains that if everything were to stay the same, this would contradict change and development.

Day-to-day work in psychotherapy confirms this view. In psychotherapy work consists also in increasing awareness, changing mindsets and behaviour. In the course of the therapeutic confrontation, people can learn to handle burdening life situations and difficulties differently and suffer less as a consequence.[200] This is often very hard work for everybody concerned. Underlying a change in mindsets are mental patterns and the interaction of daily habits plus economic, social, cultural and political structures.[201]

People in crises are more willing to try something new, instead of continuing down the same path. An open attitude in conjunction with therapeutic interventions can help people to disrupt certain destructive behavioural patterns. Irrespective of the context, whether it be within a familiar system or in social business, a crisis can bring hidden qualities to light and/or allow them to develop. The same principle applies to larger structures, although here the complexity increases.

Social entrepreneurs are good examples of how an open and flexible mental attitude can help to overcome difficult phases constructively. The researcher Froma Walsh found that, put simply, the worst times in a person's life can bring out the best.[202] Resilience research shows that it is possible to discover the good in difficult situations.[203] People with resilience maintain hope despite problematic circumstances. A crisis can contribute towards a person taking unsuspected new directions, seek change and increase his or her mental flexibility.

Social entrepreneurs experience fixed mindsets as the largest obstacles for realising their visions. Boxed-in attitudes are typical of institutions, organizations and structures whose image of the world and of people are rigid or who live in "prisons of imagination"[204] as Goetz Werner put so appropriately. Social entrepreneurs consider mindsets and the challenge of trying to change them as the most difficult obstacle in realizing social visions.

6.2 Lack of Trust

Helpers and practioners in various fields of work (psycho-social, educational etc.) sometimes have too little faith in the capabilities of people in crises to develop and find solutions to their problems themselves. Some social entrepreneurs believe that this lack of faith and trust in the potential of those in need hinders sustainability. Although those in need receive something by the support provided, something is also taken away from them stated Alisa del Tufo on the basis of her many years of experience:

"One of the other divisions in our country and maybe in yours too, is that professionals have so little trust of people who have problems, as if they have no ability to solve their problems. They may need encouragement, support, resources, but they actually know how to solve their own problems, except for extreme cases. But we take so much of that away from people. I feel as if that's a revolution that needs to happen to really find different ways of working to address our problems."[205]

Prevention in the health and social sectors need community-based, effective ways to jointly master the dynamics. The mainstream of support systems today are still miles away from this approach.

A stronger holistically orientated attitude towards help and support should become more integrated in the thoughts of politicians and decision makers. That would put us in a better position to face the immense challenges ahead.

6.3 Time

The biggest challenge for human civilization, according to Marco Roveda, is time. He wonders whether, in view of the global environmental problems, there is enough time for our awareness to make the necessary changes to be able to survive. He reminds us that part of the world's population is continually dying from famine, in armed conflicts, wars and so on. Time is quoted as a challenge in other contexts, too. One of the interview partners stated that people want everything immediately. This is often not possible. Investors want to see rapid results. But results need time, particularly when addressing social problems.

For some social entrepreneurs a further challenge are the needs of their own children who want to spend more time with them. They find that it helps to explain to the children what they are trying to do. In this way they can understand the absence of their parents better.

6.4 Financial Issues

For most of interview partners financial issues were a subject of discussion. They experience the need to guarantee the financial vitality of their social business as a continuous challenge. The start-up phase particularly and the time it requires to reach financial vitality is often long and difficult. For some, maintaining financial vitality remains a constant theme. It uses up a lot of time which they would prefer to invest in their core business. Earl Marthin Phalen says:

"Those early years were definitely challenging. That's why I said, it goes back to why you are doing this. I think most organizations go under because the leadership can't withstand the pressure of getting through that start-up-phase." The first few years feel like a learning phase. Some social businesses also lack a business plan.

and:

"There are high quality results for children and so you say, how do you do that, part of it is having a business model that actually is scalable, which I think lot of us in the nonprofit sector miss. We get passion about the idea and then we say oh the money stuff, we have to raise it, but really coming up with the business model that scales as you grow, that's been one of the big lessons."[206]

On top of that, the financing of prevention and sustainable work has become tougher, as economic global turbulences have made finding sponsors more difficult. What follows is a reduction of the scope of the business to crisis intervention and emergency programmes only. Social entrepreneurs often have to lobby intensely, especially at a stage where there is hardly any sign of success yet. It takes a lot of time to generate this money and diverts resources from the core work. For several social entrepreneurs, financial survival and gaining financial stability does not come easy, as they are not in the profit business. Still, income has to be generated and this requires innovation. The material survival is a challenge for some.

One dilemma of social entrepreneurs is the fact that the stakeholders are often reluctant to exceed a certain business size. They fear a loss in quality of their social mission. They think you cannot be good and big at the same time.

Investors could be shy to invest in social business because they see the social sector as less profitable than other sectors. Here increased efforts need to be made e.g. to communicate the social benefits more clearly. Ashoka has shown too that some social entrepreneurs pay too little attention to clearly communicating the social benefits of what they are doing.[207] This can hamper financing. In Austria, the NPO Competence Center of the Vienna University of Economics and Business is analyzing Social Return on Investment (SROI).[208]

Thomas Druyen defines wealth culture as "[…] the nurturing and maintenance of material and immaterial values, of relationships and networks to protect the individual, familiar, social and global sustainability."[209] Social entrepreneurs implement this principle by applying profit-orientated concepts. The profit generated is reinvested into the social business to help it have a larger impact.

6.5 Corruption

Social entrepreneurs need to deal with the global virus of corruption, too, which infiltrates all parts of society. They sometimes find it hard to decide which investments can be made, which offers from stakeholders are ethical and can be accepted and which have to be refused. Some of them also find it hard to find suitable people (team, advisors, successors).

Bill Drayton assumes that one reason for the increase in corruption could be that old mechanisms dealing with penalties and rewards have become less effective. Now there is more focus on the integrity of individuals and their personal values. Those responsible need to maintain integrity despite the seductive opportunities around and in the absence of any penalties and rewards.[210]

Gloria de Souza is particularly saddened by the fact that corruption is commonplace in the education sector. One of the many effects of that is that many children cannot get good school education without the high additional costs of private tuition. Many cannot afford this, although they would like to offer good quality education to their children.

"But the most heartbreaking thing, that I find it difficult to come to terms with, that the rich get richer and the poor get poorer. While India is now been seen as a country that is making a lot of progress, there is a lot of wealth. But how can you call that wealth, when it is not distributed? It echoes the sadness of a lot of people who are saying, yes probably betrayed our founding father, there is increasing corruption at all levels I feel. Pick-pockets are beaten up and thrown in jail. What is their crime, compared to all the teachers for instance, who don't teach properly in class so that after school they can make a big income, they are encouraging the fact that good teaching is not taking place during class time, so that people pay extra." (Note: for private tuition in the afternoon)"[211]

Social entrepreneurs sometimes find it hard to determine where limits to financial dependency need to be drawn and which advisors can be trusted.

In summary all social entrepreneurs face many obstacles and difficulties, go through phases of frustration, hardship and annoyances. Some find it hard to keep up their sense of purpose as their business grows and becomes more successful, when they need to deal more and more with administration, moving them further away from providing direct service to people. One social entrepreneur says that here it is vital to take care, to reenergize oneself: "How to feed your soul."[212]

Even in the course of speaking about the challenges, some already start to think about possible solutions. They reflect on what they personally could do differently. Their optimism is obvious by the way they speak. An important component of their success is the way they face challenges and difficulties (ESSE), as described above.

7. Conclusion

Formative experiences and the strong emotions associated with them plus the unswerving will to bring about changes which are good and constructive are important elements for the success (ESSE) of the social entrepreneurs and social business personalities.[213] They support others in need, are actively engaged in the protection of the environment and try to contribute to more social justice.

The fundament for their motivation is a strong set of values which withstands heavy mental shocks and which is connected to the ability to actively turn to others to tap into a variety of material and immaterial resources (ESSE).

These social entrepreneurs have a high level of self awareness and are well aware of their personal limits (ESSE). They combine their business skills, including looking for possibilities, grabbing chances, willingness to take risks, creativity and perseverance with a deeply engrained sense of social responsibility. This gives them the core motivation to do what they do (ESSE). Another thing which has become apparent throughout the study is that sustainable social business is possible in any cultural context.

For psychotherapeutic practice and research it is clear that resilient elements and salutogenesis have large value for the support of health. An even greater paradigm shift is needed where more focus is placed on the healthy and less on the pathological. This may sound paradoxical as people usually seek therapy when they are ill and suffer. So it seems reasonable that the suffering is the focus, but it is more helpful if this is practised only to a certain extend in order people feel understood and their suffering is recognized. Or to put it into Steve de Shazers [214] words: "Energy flows where attention goes."

Summarizing the results of my scientific analyses which have provided the basis for this publication: they clearly show how the personalities succeed, despite adverse conditions, and manage to lead a healthy, fulfilling life.[215] These aspects should be integrated into teachings and practice a lot more (ESSE).

8. Outlook

Through their actions, all social entrepreneurs that were interviewed have had a concrete beneficial impact on the well-being of many people. The experiences and motivations of the social business personalities and their elements of success (ESSE) is the focus of this book. They faced and succeeded challenges such as doing away with mechanistic ways of thinking, developing a stronger orientation towards both individual and collective sustainability and holistic mindsets. A rethink in many areas, both in practice and theory is necessary and would be forward-thinking. This includes, the educational sector and vocational training. Fortunately this is already happening to some extent and a transition is already underway.[216]

One-sided (often one-sidedly interpreted) theories are unsustainable, both individually and collectively. This is true for many sectors, for instance the health sector where prevention in health care still has a relatively low priority compared to the treatment of symptoms.[217] In the economic sector, the maximization of material profits is still the basis for many actions without taking other possible impacts into account, such as the social benefit or the Social Return (SROI).[218]

In the face of global crises and economic crises in particular, preventive interventions, projects and also psychotherapy can help to reduce, relieve or even cure mental suffering, including depressions and burn-out resulting from unhealthy working conditions. This would, as a whole, have a positive effect on (health and other) budgets of governments and countries and would reduce economic costs substantially. Everybody, especially some responsible, need to make an effort to create more humane working conditions and relations, implementing values such as creating meaning in the work, for everybody concerned.

Social entrepreneurial skills, engaging oneself for the common good and the elements to succeed can be promoted both in children and in grown-ups (ESSE). A holistic education could start as early as elementary school. Lessons of empathy,[219] self-responsibility, creativity and the search for support could be reinforced and introduced on a larger scale, such as extending it to university education. This requires the engagement and courage of those responsible, of teachers in various disciplines, parents, active students and other stakeholders. This may sound utopian, but history has often shown that ideas, which originally seemed utopian, can be implemented successfully. An historic example is the introduction of systems of social security in Europe.

If we are seriously interested and there is a good will, if interdisciplinary and intersectoral cooperation is the true concern, it will be possible to provide targeted support of the elements leading to success (ESSE) in many areas.[220] Synergies can be achieved on all sides. The results would be multi-dimensional and would have a wide-ranging positive impact on the health of many.

Appendix

For the interested reader:

Our Personality and its Many Faces

There is no standard definition for the term "personality". It depends on the current Zeitgeist, on worldviews and conceptions of man. Related to it are the terms "character" and "person" which are derived etymologically from the Greek where their original meaning was character in the widest sense. The term "character" refers to the shaped individuality.[221] "Personality" on the other hand is described as a unique system of characteristics of a person which has developed through his or her individual biography. It is controlled according to the situation and consolidates itself in the course of his or her life.[222] Here I would like to note though that this concept of "consolidation", as mentioned in the encyclopaedia,[223] has been disproven by science and by the experiences made in psychotherapeutic practice. Elderly people for instance are well able to change decade-old habits or make utterly life-changing decisions.

In the academic world the term "character" was gradually replaced by the term "personality". Some schools of depth psychology, however, still prefer the term "character", especially those which consider early childhood as the main influence on the subsequent course of life of a person.

In an interview, the psychotherapist and cultural scientist Bernd Rieken speaks about changing values and patchwork identities.[224] He highlights psychosocial and cultural aspects of the human personality and puts them into the context of the enormous processes of individualization dominating western cultural societies. Modern day life in western societies has many advantages. People can develop and express their individuality in many different ways. Fundamental decisions are made individually, including the choice of partner, education, job and where and how to live. This freedom of choice as lived in modern western societies is relatively new historically and is not a matter of course in many other cultures and parts of the world.

Throughout human history this extent and type of freedom was unknown and can be considered a large step in societal development. Whilst it certainly is an achievement, it also brings about new psychological challenges for the individual. In the absence of given structures, which she or he can grow into, people in western societies need to seek, form and develop a substantial part of their orientation, standards for action and way of life themselves.[225] So to a certain extent life has become more complicated and sometimes the demands on the individual can become too much.

Out of my practical experience in psychotherapy and mediation, added to this are the social expectations and/or the desire of the individual to lead a different life to that of the parents. This is a large challenge for mothers and fathers when raising children.

Fortunately our aim is to provide our children with the best childhood possible. It is widely assumed that the lion's share of their development happens through education. At the same time there is pressure on parents to look after their own personal development, too, both privately and professionally. This is a lot to handle. The huge amount of information and advice on child education available now only helps to a limited degree and sometimes even contradicts itself in central questions. On top of that most parents have experienced the frustration of having limited emotional resources, for instance when trying to deal with their strong-willed child, realizing that their son or daughter is much harder to influence than what the literature suggests.[226] This can result in an increase in personal pressure and give rise to feelings of guilt, anger etc. towards the child. The effects of this can be the perception of being a failure, anxiety disorders, a decreased feeling of self-worth and feelings of insecurity. In individualistic societies the individual bears responsibility for how she or he leads his or her life. As a consequence she or he is also responsible for failure. In traditionalistic societies responsibility and blame are shared more than in individualistic societies. In the latter, the wide gap between our self image and our aim, between the "can, should, must" and what we actually experience can be substantial. The increase of such pressures can contribute to the rise in mental illnesses, such as depression, anxiety disorders, burn-out etc.[227]

According to Rieken, the scientific community sees the human character as being influenced by environmental factors on the one hand and genetic factors on the other. A third factor is the ego identity of a person.[228] The ego identity is particularly relevant from the point of view of psychotherapy.

Throughout history, human beings have always been interested in looking for explanations for human experiences and behaviour. Rieken quotes the ancient Greeks, whose scientific view of the human being was greatly influenced by the humoral medicine which assumes that the human character is formed by external factors.[229] This theory of the human temperaments is amongst the oldest attempts to characterize people. It distinguishes four basic types which are defined by bodily fluids: the sanguine type who has a lot of temperament (blood), the lethargic, slow phlegmatic type (mucus), the constantly worrying melancholy type (black gall) and the choleric type (yellow gall) who is irritable and prone to impulsive behaviour. This theory has become part of everyday language. Occasionally clients of psychotherapy classify themselves on the basis of this theory, or else their family and friends do. In therapy, some clients are confronted with their own deterministic view that the temperament and the associated state of mind "is formed once and for all". This is clearly not the case. Otherwise humans would not be able to develop (see also resilience) and psychotherapy would make little sense. Science and practice prove that change is possible.

Other long outdated theories also continue to influence people. This has an effect on decisions in social policy, education, jurisdiction and health care to name just a few areas. The question as to whether a person can change is fundamental for insurance companies. Is it worth supporting psychotherapy as part of health care? The answer to this question is still influenced by the traditional ways of thinking of the decision-makers.

Personality models usually differ in the following aspects:[230]

- to what extent the personality is made up of relatively static characteristics (particularly with early explanations of personality)
- to what extent environmental factors shape the personality;
- how much they refer to measurable data and facts; and
- whether subconscious components are part of a personality and to what extent.

In the following some theories on personality are briefly outlined. They illustrate the different ways of thinking. They include theories on general mental patterns which enable a comparison of people as well as theories on the inner structures of a person, defining his or her uniqueness. Some of these theories supported the interpretation of some of the aspects of the social entrepreneurs I interviewed.

1. Psychodynamic Models

Psychodynamic models include psychoanalysis as developed by Sigmund Freud, but other models, too, which were developed by his pupils. Some used his theory as the basis for their own work and others distanced themselves from him and were critical of him. Alfred Adler, Carl Gustav Jung, Henry A. Murray und Erik H. Erikson were amongst them. Freud's psychoanalytical concept consists of structural factors (ego, id and super-ego), dynamic and genetic aspects (urges: sexual urge, urge for self preservation, urge to destroy, aggression; psychosexual development phases: oral, anal, phallic, latency and genital) as well as therapeutic aspects. Expressed simply, he assumed that the development of a child in becoming an adult passes various stages. If it experiences sufficient pleasure in a certain stage, it will pass on to the next stage smoothly. If it does not, a fixation will develop. On the other hand if it experiences too much pleasure in any one stage, the child will regress and remain in that stage.

Freud saw the "id" as the area of the psyche where primary, inherent, subconscious urges lie, whilst the ego represents conscious, reality orientation. The ego is a mediator between the id and the outside world. The third structural factor or area of the psyche, according to Freud, is the so-called "super-ego" which represents norms, values, moral ideas of parents, authorities and culture. Freud described human emotions and behaviour as a dynamic, an interplay between these three factors. He considered the unfolding of subconscious psychosexuality as having a substantial influence on the personality of a person and spoke about the "id" as not being master in its own house.[231]

According to Alfred Adler, our personality develops within the tension between selfishness and sense of community, where trying to overcome feelings of inferiority plays a central role.[232] Adler saw the drive to be powerful as the basic engine for human behaviour. Carl Gustav Jung divided the unconscious into an individual and collective part and considered this relevant for our personality.

Charlotte Bühler, Abraham Maslow, Carl Rogers, Erich Fromm and Viktor Frankl are representatives of humanistic approaches. To them individual fulfillment is a paramount value. Their main focus is the individual as a whole plus his or her conscious experiences.

The psychotherapist Erik H. Erikson[233] developed a model based on the psychoanalytical theory of Freud. Erikson expanded Freud's phases and divided childhood into eight psychosocial phases. As his theory is an important link for other models on personality, it shall be described in some detail in the following subchapters.

Erikson's particular interest lay in the examination of the core of an individual. However, he also highlighted social and cultural conditions and emphasised that the individual phases need to be seen as part of the whole. The separate phases are related to one of the basic components of society. Some of them are summarized below.[234]

Trust (vs. Mistrust)

A child's first social achievement is to manage to let its mother leave its field of vision by turning her into an inner certainty. In this process the child detaches itself from her as a reliably present external appearance. A first feeling of ego identity develops, "… which depends, I think, on the recognition that there is an inner population of remembered and anticipated sensations and images which are firmly correlated with the outer population of familiar and predictable things and people."[235]

Analytically, the root of particularly deep mechanisms lies in the early process of distinguishing between the inner and outer. An inner injury is transferred to an outer person who then represents the "bad" which lies within. On the other hand something good in the outer world is turned into inner certainty in the process of introjection. One of the first tasks of the ego is to meet central conflicts of trust and mistrust with certain behaviour. Trust for instance is strengthened if individual needs are met by being cared for sensitively. Trust is linked more to the quality of a relationship than to the quantity.

Erikson stated that there are only few denials a child cannot endure as long as it experiences that they strengthen its self-assurance and help to integrate it into a meaningful, larger belonging. However, Erikson believes that, even under the most favourable circumstances, "a sense of a feeling of inner division and universal nostalgia for a paradise forfeited"[236] is left in the psyche.

Autonomy (vs. Shame and Doubt)

In this second phase the child's muscular system continues to develop. This relates to the basic social component of holding on and letting go. In this stage the child needs to be lead securely and firmly without robbing it of its freedom to make decisions appropriate to its developmental stage. Erikson connects the emergence of the child's feeling of shame with its awareness of how exposed it is. All eyes are on it now. This makes it feel insecure.

According to this theory, the tendency for doubt and shame arises from the child experiencing a loss of self-control. It is aware that another person or persons have authority over it. It experiences an invasion into its autonomy and its excretion processes. Doubt arises as its excrements are suddenly considered bad by the grown ups after digestion processes had always been considered good previously. In this phase anger, jealousy and rivalry arises and can lead to assaults on the younger siblings. Feeling ashamed for something rapidly leads to a feeling of guilt.

Initiative (vs. Guilt)

With each new stage the child experiences yet another level of vitality. In this third phase it is now able to move freely and has also developed an infantile sexuality. The basic social components of this stage are the "doing" and "approaching".

Infantile sexuality, incest tabu, castration complex and the super ego all lead the child to a process of emotional reform. It develops two parts - an infantile and a parental part. The infantile part remains enthusiastic about its continuing growth. The parental part encourages self-reflection, making own decisions and punishing itself. According to Erikson, the "oedipal phase" paves the way for the development of morality, but also sows the seed for the child's reflections on what its possibilities are, how adult life might look like, tapping into its early childhood dreams.

Industry (vs. Inferiority)

In all cultures children now enter the life of the grown ups where they are systematically taught a variety of things, be it in nature, on the street or in the classroom. They learn to use different everyday things and tools e.g. they learn how to read and write, the basis for a future choice of profession. Usually a child only has a vague idea of the roles of her or his mother and father. This is a consequence of the complexity of social reality. In this fourth phase, feelings of inferiority and inadequacy can start to grow. This phase is socially relevant, as what counts now is "to perform", especially with regard to others.

Identity (vs. Role Confusion)

This phase marks the end of childhood. Puberty commences and the earlier urges emerge, dominated by the adolescent's genitality. How she or he is seen by others becomes important. Erikson describes the adolescent mind as being in a psychological stage between child and adulthood. It is an ideological mind which has to find her or his place between the ethical values learnt and those which need to be developed as a young adult. Social values are actively sought as orientation for the adolescent's own identity.

Intimacy (vs. Isolation)

According to Erikson, the body and ego now need to overcome the core conflicts and master the organ modalities to be able to surrender to someone or something without being afraid of losing the ego. Surrender is needed during orgasm, sexual union, in close friendship, in physical conflicts as well as in moments of inspiration by teachers and mentors and intuition. A person will often try to avoid such experiences, avoid intimacy to prevent the feared loss of the ego. The consequence is a feeling of isolation and a predominant occupation with oneself.

The full development of the so-called true genitality is important. It adds a feeling of ethics into sex. Ideally this leads to a complete sharing of emotions with a beloved partner and the aim to try to harmonize the various parts of life, such as work and recuperation.

Generativity (vs. Stagnation)

The term "generativity" describes productivity and creativity and the interest to pass on knowledge to the next generation.[237] To surrender to the union of body and soul leads to a gradual expansion of the interests of the ego and to joyful creation. Generativity is a fundamental phase of the psychosexual and psychosocial development plan. It should be noted that generativity does not necessarily include reproduction and offspring.

Ego Integrity (vs. Despair)

Erikson describes ego integrity as a phase of increasing certainty with regard to our order and purpose. A sense of purpose is now felt, irrespective of what the "price" was. He speaks of the need to accept our individual and unique path through life. This changes our relationship to our parents:

"Although aware of the relativity of all the various life styles which have given meaning to human striving, the possessor of integrity is ready to defend the dignity of his own style against all physical and economic threats."[238]

Erikson explains that each civilization uses a particular combination of conflicts for the development of a particular style of integration. What he means is that infantile conflicts become creative conflicts if they find safe ground in society's cultural institutions or in its representatives. He writes:

"[…] (1) that the human personality in principle develops according to steps predetermined in the growing person's readiness to be driven towards, to be aware of, and to interact with, a widening social radius; and (2) that society, in principle, tends to be so constituted as to meet and invite this succession of potentialities for interaction and attempts to safeguard and to encourage the proper rate and the proper sequence of their enfolding." [239]

Erikson points out that his model does not represent a scale of achievement. For instance, gaining trust is not an achievement which is secured once and for all. This specific note of Erikson receives too little attention in various psychotherapeutic concepts. Accepting it would weaken some of the claims of feasibility in psychotherapeutic practice.

Erikson explains that negative sentiments (for instance basic mistrust) remain the active opposite sides of positive sentiments throughout a person's life. He cautions that his model should not be misunderstood. Each of the phases goes through expansion and crisis before it arrives at a solution:

"But they all must exist from the beginning in some form, for every act calls for an integration of all. Also, an infant may show something like 'autonomy' from the beginning in the particular way in which he angrily tries to wriggle himself free when tightly held." [240]

Each psychosocial achievement is accompanied by a core conflict which strengthens the young person by providing him or her with an additional new quality. The young person experiences the "whole critical opposition of being an autonomous creature and being a dependent one" [241] and prepares him or herself to face it. Erikson considers it a culture's contribution to the health of a human personality by the way it communicates autonomy and rules.

Erikson adds the following values to his explanations. They are hardly anchored in his theoretical model. One reason for this might be the hurdles he may have encountered whilst researching them. For example in his efforts to examine the concept of fidelity, he came across methodical hurdles.

He defines the qualities listed below as the lasting result of favourable conditions:

- "Basic Trust v. Basic Mistrust: Drive and *Hope*
- Autonomy v. Shame and Doubt: Self-Control and *Willpower*
- Initiative v. Guilt: Direction and *Purpose*
- Industry v. Inferiority: Method and *Competence*
- Identity v. Role Confusion: Devotion and *Fidelity*
- Intimacy v. Isolation: Affiliation and *Love*
- Generativity v. Stagnation: Production and *Care*
- Ego Integrity v. Despair: Renunciation and *Wisdom*."[242]

In conclusion, according to Erikson the personality can continue to develop throughout one's lifetime. He emphasises that the virtues are essential as without them all other human value systems would lose their meaning and relevance.

In the next chapters further models which played a role in interpreting my research results are discussed.

2 Systemics

There is no uniform systems theory, just as little as there is a classical personality theory within the various systems theories as they focus mainly on relationships and on context issues.

Günter Schiepek,[243] suggests that the reason for the lack of a uniform systems theory could be the fact that systemic thinking developed relatively independently from a diversity of disciplines including biology, physics, chemistry, ecology, sociology, philosophy a.o. Etymologically the root of the word *system* lies in the Greek where *systema* means a composition of elements forming a superordinate entity which is greater than the sum of its parts. In the 1950ies the development of various systemic theories began in the natural sciences, in economics, and later on also in the areas of therapy and sociology. Following this, system theory was applied to other areas, too. The mediator and psychotherapist Joseph Duss-von Werdt stated: "As part of the whole itself, the human being is not all. But in interacting with other parts of the whole it forms larger or smaller systems with them."[244]

Relationships between people and between phenomena

are the core focus of systemic thinking. Viewed traditionally, people "have" certain qualities, whilst in systemic thinking these qualities only surface in relation to the characteristics of others. In other words they are context dependant. Here is an example to illustrate this: in class a certain girl is hyperactive and transgressive. The behaviour of the same girl changes completely when she goes for a walk with her aunt. Viewed systemically, the behaviour of the child is dependent on which situation she is in and with which people. Viewed from this perspective, each figure has a background. Another important aspect is language. Several researchers, including Bateson et al and the Humberto Maturana who examined the phenomenon of recognition concluded: "Everything said is said by someone."[245] These researchers consider language as the tool of recognition and note that it is its problem at the same time.

The systemic perspective focuses on interpersonal phenomena. Particularly in the early days of systemic therapy development, practitioners and scientists came from different theoretical backgrounds with different concepts on personal identity. Helm Stierlin, a systemic therapist of the early days states the following with regard to identity: "Such a feeling of identity is both the expression and consequence of a permanent construction of a self which only seems possible if temporal and situative contexts are ignored."[246] A few efforts were made to integrate the concepts of personal identity and self within systemic therapy theories.[247] Two examples of this are summarized in the following.

Dialectics of the Personality[248]

Helmut Johnson was missing a holistic theory on man and nature[249] and addressed the scientific development of a systemically orientated theory on personality in his "Dialectics of the Personality". He considers the personality as the dialectic unit of a historic programme and its real behaviour. With "historic programmes" Johnson means the family of origin whose potential may often be unavailable, but who is still there. The interaction with others is a necessary prerequisite and condition for personal development. Individuality cannot develop in isolation. Consequently Johnson insists that when considering the character of a person the "history as identified via the family and which is contained in everything"[250] has to be included.

PSI-Theorie[251]

Julius Kuhl developed a theory of Personality-System-Interactions (PSI Theory) which illustrates how a person's system of insights works. The PSI theory can be combined with theories on the social and cultural context. Kuhl integrates the hypotheses of various personality theories and findings of experimental psychology and neurobiology to form a system with which he attempts explain human behaviour. According to Kuhl, the activation of mental systems as well as the exchange of information between them is dependent on moods and the emotion at the moment. He assumes that people who have learnt how to deal with their feelings in their child-hood can activate the type of "mental system" they need at the moment, such as the ability to regulate fear and anger. On a positive note the author integrates aspects of various personality theories, which have received less at-tention so far, such as forms of intuition and spirituality. However, with Kuhl's assumption that mental systems are "retrievable" he introduces a factor of control into the theory which could seem incompatible with these dimensions.

The PSI Theory refers to analytic-explicit and holis-tic-intuitive forms of insight. Kuhl sees a mature person as someone who develops plans and sets targets with which she or he can identify herself or himself with and which harmonize with own needs and values as well as with the social environment. This approach agrees with that of Carl Gustav Jung[252] and Ken Wilber,[253] amongst others, who integrated the aspect of spirituality into their theories.[254] These approaches have often been and still are ignored by experimental psychology and by theories which are reduced to considering mainly the biology of a human.

Jung hoped that research on the various personality types would lead to an increased appreciation of how different we all are, thus contributing to a peaceful co-existence.

Systemic approaches focus mainly on relationships and interactions and on the context and not on the aspect of identity. Apart from that, they contain aspects of salu-togenesis, as described in the following chapter.

3 Salutogenesis

Salutogenesis is a preventative concept for supporting and maintaining personal health. It was developed by Aaron Antonovsky, a professor of medical sociology. The trigger to the development of his concept were his research results which strikingly illustrated the relatively good mental and physical health of the survivors of Nazi concentration camps despite the incredible tortures they had experienced. He tackled the question of how health develops and realized that health is not a condition but a development. Thomas Druyen, describes health as the necessary basis for our mental and productive wealth.[255] Responsibility for our own life style consists of looking after our health and protecting it with measures provided by the State and private institutions.[256] According to Antonovsky, the central element supporting health is a "sense of coherence" (SOC). This SOC means that a person, irrespective of culture, has a deep feeling of trust that life's challenges can be met.[257] Depending on the extent of the SOC health can develop.

The focus shifts from suffering and pathology to looking for chances and opportunities.[258] For instance symptoms such as stomach pains can be an indication of stress. A person experiencing this symptom has the chance to work on his or her stress factors to reduce them. For Antonovsky these chances provide the potential for the development of health. Health and illness are influenced both by the individual experience and independent conditions. Everybody is equipped with healthy and sick parts. He refers to the multi-dimensionality of the health process and points out how it relates to the cultural and social environment.

A point of critique: Antonovsky states that the development of a sense of coherence is completed at around 25 years of age. That would mean that this ability cannot be strengthened or improved in a person beyond that age, such as for instance via psychotherapy.[259] This aspect contradicts his thought of health as a continuous process.

4 Resilience

Resilience is the ability of a person to use difficult situations in his or her life for personal development by including both personal and social resources. Despite the challenges met mental health is maintained or even improved. Resilience is a process which does not ignore stress and dangers, but enables a person to deal with these factors in a beneficial way. The ability to actively face challenges, plus the cultural, the family and wider social environment influence the process.

Emmy E. Werner und Ruth Smith undertook research on aspects of resilience decades ago:[260] a long-term study of 698 children who had been born on the Hawaiian island of Kauai in 1955. All of these children had been exposed to risk factors, more than a third of them to high risk factors. Werner and Smith's research results showed that the development of more than a third of the high risk children proceeded remarkably positively.[261] They turned into healthy, trustworthy and competent adults. The researchers identified several protective factors which helped the participants. These included a stable emotional relationship to a person outside of the family, active participation within the community, being embedded in a community of faith and a high internal "locus of control".[262] The participants made the experience that they could influence their own fate and that their own behaviour and actions had real consequences. Other practitioners and scientists dealing with resilience include Michael Rutter,[263] Nathan Caplan,[264] Rosemarie Welter-Enderlin,[265] Jens Asendorpf[266] and Friedrich Lösel.[267]

Lösel and his co-workers arrived at similar conclusions with respect to protective factors. They studied 144 children who were brought up in homes. Resilient people not only endure and survive adverse conditions, but also tap into hitherto unknown resources in extreme situations. Bruno Hildebrand also speaks of attributes which support resilience and provides a description of the process. According to him, resilience is an expression of a specific type of orientation and action.[268] Sir Michael Rutter highlights the process character of resilience: adaptive versus maladaptive coping can be a reaction to a challenge. The definition of the experience which is felt as a crisis plays a role here.[269] Findings from research on resilience are turned into practice in some parts of the United States of Amerika. Children in elementary school are taught key elements of resilience:

"Look for a friend and be a friend to others. Take responsibility for your actions. Believe in yourself." [270]

This training needs to be carefully adapted to the developmental stages of the child, though, as otherwise excessive demands might be made on it. For instance the child may not be in a position to change a difficult situation. In this case placing large emphasis on its individual responsibility may increase its fear of failure and reduce its feeling of self-worth.

Rosmarie Welter-Enderlin organised a conference on "resilience" in Zürich in 2005 in quoting Albert Camus: "In the midst of winter I realized that there is an unconquerable summer within me". Welter-Enderlin und Werner summarise: "The assumption that a child from a high risk family will inevitably become a loser is disproved by the research on resilience."[271]

Approaches tending towards resilience contain important systemic elements as they move away from the pathological and move towards salutogenesis. This does not mean that all we need to do is to look for resources. That would be too simplistic, also it would suggest that people can do much more than they actually can.

5 Cultural Aspects

The social entrepreneurs I interviewed live in various parts of the world and come from a variety of different cultural backgrounds.[272] The term "culture", as applied here, is a dynamic and evolving one. Only occasionally territorial aspects are included, if they are relevant. This interpretation ties in with modern social anthropology.

Heidi Schär Sall and her co-workers[273] no longer define culture by ethnic groups or by territory. They emphasise

"[…] the increasing complexity in the sense of merging processes of translocal and global contexts. Culture is interpreted more and more as a negotiation process of meanings […].The question of culture therefore is the question of the various, constantly changing constructions of the worlds of meaning of an invidual within the context of his or her life-style."[274]

The increasing diversity of societies in the globalised world can be enriching. On the other hand it can also sharpen existing conflicts and create new ones, namely between the society of origin and the receiving society. This development is apparent in health care, so also in psychotherapy. Here too, we observe how different values and interpretations of health and illness are.[275] Depending on the background and setting, communication of the various interpretations is essential.

Schär Sall sees a danger in

"[…] not recognizing and supporting factors of resilience due to our own ethnocentrism, in fact even devaluing them. For instance, the rapid changing of relationships with high social flexibility which represented an important survival strategy of a patient may be interpreted as an attachment disorder. Often significant social dynamics and their stable relationships can only be recognized when looking at the extended group. Understanding different models of socialization and their invidual and collective implications is of paramount importance with regard to resilience factors. In fact people with a different socialization often come into conflict with the rigid expectation of a highly structured society and its institutions.

This rigidity can be experienced as "persecuting", leading to aggressive transferences on both sides, if it remains not understood."[276]

In psychotherapeutic practice, cross-cultural aspects are taken into consideration to be able to understand people and their personal set of values. For this reason the question of resilience is significant in psychotherapy, particularly within the context of vulnerability. Here there is room for a lot of research and for a change in mindsets.

6 Emotions

Luc Ciompi has been studying the structure of the psyche, inner and outer worlds, feelings, affects and the emotional fundaments of human thinking for many years.[277] His concept is based on Freud, his own psychiatric and psychotherapeutic experiences and on significant findings of system theory, neurobiology and psycho- and sociodynamics. He emphasises that "modern brain research shows that, functionally, centres of thought and feeling are inseparable and constantly influence each other intensely."[278] Ciompi defines "affects" as the psycho-somatic state of a person whereby the duration and degree of consciousness is variable. The author qualifies: " (…) scientifically at least we only know very vaguely what a feeling is, what the sense of it is and how it works."[279] He uses fear as an example, an energetic state geared towards flight. Or he describes how joy or love affect the entire body.

According to Ciompi, science avoided the concepts of feelings, emotions and affects and their relevance to conceptions of man and world views for a long time, as these phenomena are not easily understood, are irrational and often unpleasant. As a consequence there was a tendency towards one sided conceptions and views composed of so-called "objective" thoughts and insights. In recent years an "emotional turning point" has become apparent as countermovement to the "cognitive" turning point. Gradually the theories of behaviourism of the sixties of the past century are being replaced.[280]

Ciompi groups his findings into five theories. He calls them affect logic. This means that feelings, emotions and affects have an influence on every event, including the daily incidents in families, jobs and politics, bursts of violence, revolutions and wars.[281] Other specialists and people who make use of their experiences and perceptions share this opinion, for instance Bernd Rieken notes: "Feelings have an influence on everything we do."[282] Ciompi's definition of affect also includes the energetic dimension and the intention, in other words the motivational aspect. Part of this is illustrated in the following chapter.

7 Conscious or unconscious?

According to Gottfried Fischer, unconscious intentionality plays a role in human interactions.[283] In psychotherapy, there is the unanimous opinion that subconsciously motivated behaviour exists and that the term is not a contradiction in itself.

Fischer has been researching this phenomenon and the problem of recognising it. Depending on how well behaviour and motive fit together, behaviour can provide an indication of a motive.[284] Recurring behavioural patterns can also be an indication of unconscious motives, particularly if the behaviour is in discrepancy with the situation experienced. Another indicator for unconscious motives is the extent to which the own self image and behaviour of affected persons change once they recognize their own contradictions. Fischer emphasises that unconscious intentional behaviour is only part of unconscious behaviour and that automatisms are common, too.

He clarifies several frequent misunderstandings between biological psychiatry, experimental psychology and psychotherapy. He refers for instance to the assumption of some representatives of biological psychiatry and neurology that our thoughts and decisions are driven purely by physico-chemical process. He argues that this is presumptive, as there is no empirical evidence.[285]In merely considering physico-chemical aspects, the psycho-social processes of our human existence are ignored.

He argues that research results need to be translated back into the everyday context. He criticizes that the deduced "ideal constructions" of natural science are often wrongly seen as the "true reality".[286] Adopting the philosopher Bieri's thoughts on the relative freedom of will, he illustrates the following:

"Imagine a delinquent defending himself in court arguing that not he himself planned and carried out the crime, but his brain did. No court in the world would content itself with this. Many consider scientific constructions as the true reality if they are abstracted from the context of everyday life. They shy away from translating them back into the context of their everyday experience, thereby 'demystifying' them."[287]

Using the example of the human freedom of will, Fischer critically examines restrictive scientific observations.

Theories should not be maintained for their own sake.[288] If they have to be rejected, because they have proven wrong, courage is needed to do so. Humberto Maturana for instance advocates that the right to change one's opinion should be defined as an additional human right.[289]Maybe the duty or right to reject theories, which have been proven false or are harmful, should become such a human right, too (see also principle of falsification; Sir Karl Popper).

E.g. Economic theories which are unsustainable for humans and the environment in the long run continue to be taught to this day. Sometimes theories are implemented in a manner which was not originally intended by those that developed them.

Within system orientated psychotherapy, the context

of how a symptom or illness began is central. Diagnostic dialogues aim at understanding this context as it is hoped that here important information for the reduction and cure of the problem will be found. Similar "interventions" could support the "health" of the "ill" economic system. For instance when theories are taught, it would be valuable if the original intentions behind them and the context within which they were developed received more attention.[290] This could lead to more flexibility in their application, more suited to the social and cultural environment in question.

During a lecture Colin Crouch held in Vienna, he criticized scientists and practitioners who propagate the concept of unlimited growth in a limited world.[291] In spite of the global economic crisis of 2008 and other proven facts, many people, including quite a few in functions of responsibility for society and politics, business people and corporations continue to cling on to the idea of unlimited growth. A possible explanation for this common behaviour apart from greed is that most people tend to want to keep up comforts and standards of living. This is understandable. They are thus not willing to change their way of thinking. It is easier to subscribe to the illusion that limitless growth is possible, despite undeniable facts such as the limited availability of our (environmental) resources.[292] One reason for this phenomenon can be human idleness.

Another example illustrates the above: various industries, including some within the health sector, refer to so-called clear evidence and use it as the basis for their marketing and sales with the aim of profit maximization. The statements made by a medical specialist at a congress on "Humanism in Medicine" is noted here.[293] She reminds that there is no lack of scientific evidence on the effectiveness of psychotherapy as treatment of illness.

Luc Ciompi found that

"there is no such thing as pure thinking, free of affects. It simply cannot exist – neither in science, nor in formal logic, not even in mathematics."[294]

He also notes that the consequences of this have not yet been adequately understood by many. One would have to agree, to a certain extent, in the face of current social, economic and political dynamics on the global and individual scale. A pressing question is: what consequences would an extended understanding have on the individual and social level?

At the end of this chapter on various aspects of the human personality and the various approaches towards researching it, I would like to quote a statement made by Jens Asendorpf, who is a personality psychologist and was a researcher at the Humboldt University in Berlin and the Max Planck Institute. After many years of research he concluded:

"There are zero correlations between the neurophysiological level and the observed or self-perceived personality. The impression is always made that neurophysiology is where we should be looking for how personality develops. However, neurophysiological parameters could just as well be caused by the different behaviour of people.

[…] If they behave in a certain way, their neuroatanomy could change, too."[295]

He emphasises that the personality is not formed and stabilized as much in the first years of childhood as numerous theories suggest. Environmental and societal effects do not play that significant a role. Asendorpf criticizes that the factor "early childhood" is rated far too highly by the classic theories. Humans are not determined to that extent. He supports his statements by several meta analyses which have been undertaken. Their results agree with important insights of research on resilience.

'The whole is more than a sum of its parts' – this popular systemic principle can also be applied to the way a personality has evolved.

References and Notes

Chapter 1

1   Amongst various ideas taken into consideration I decided to choose the one of focussing on the elements of success, which was generated by Mr. Angelantonio Ferrandina. Director of I.A.M.S. Registered Mediator (Federal Justice Ministry). Licensed Social and Life Counsellor, LifeCoach, Artist.

2   which was finalized in 2013.

3   Austrian Federal Ministry of Health: Professional Code for Psychotherapists (last version 2012). Dep. II/A/3; Legal matters - medical doctors, psychology, psychotherapy and music therapy. Paragraph VII, p. 16. The professional code requires that psychotherapists also concern themselves with themes of social relevance. "As part of their social responsibility, members of the profession of psychotherapy are required to contribute to maintaining and creating living conditions which serve to support, conserve and restore human mental health, maturation and development."

See Kierein Michael, Pritz Alfred, Sonneck Gernot (1991). Psychologen-Gesetz, Psychotherapie-Gesetz (Law on Psychology, Law on Psychotherapy). Kurzkommentar (short commentary). Orac: Vienna. p. 118ff. The Austrian Law on Psychotherapy and the ethical guidelines describe the professional obligations.

See also the Statement of Ethical Principles of the European Association of Psychotherapists (EAP), 2002, revised 2010. p. 1: "They (the psychotherapists) are committed to increasing knowledge of human behaviour and of people's understanding of themselves and others and the utilisation of such knowledge for the promotionof human welfare."

4 ibid. Thomas Druyen, sociologist and professor of comparative culture and psychology of wealth at the Sigmund Freud University (SFU) in Vienna: within the context of a talk on the topic of social business (amongst others) at the SFU on May 14, 2009 and notes on the author's presentation of the concept of this study on May 28, 2010.

5 See Achleitner, Heister, Stahl, 2007, p. 10.

6 See Interview # 9.

7 See http://oesterreich.orf.at [14. 5. 2010]; see article on OECD-Studie in: Der Standard of March 6, 2015: „Psychisch Kranke massiv von Jobverlust bedroht."

8 See Kierein Michael, Pritz Alfred, Sonneck Gernot (1991). Psychologen-Gesetz, Psychotherapie-Gesetz (Law on Psychology, Law on Psychotherapy). Kurzkommentar (short commentary). Orac: Vienna. p. 118ff. The Austrian Law on Psychotherapy and the ethical guidelines describe the professional obligations.

9 See EU-Studie of 5. 9. 2011: „The size and burden of mental disorders and other disorders of the brain in Europe." 2010, www.psychologischehochschule Berlin.de [6. 11. 2011];

An EU study on mental illnesses lead by the Dresden psychologist Hans-Ulrich Wittchen found that 38,2 % of all EU citizens suffer from this type of illness. Also, substantial shortcomings in the treatment of patients were found, as therapies often started late and only around a third of those affected actually received treatment.

See also WHO prognosis of global extent for 2020;

10 See http://oesterreich.orf.at [14. 5. 2010]. Europewide campaign supported by the European and Austrian networks for workplace health promotion and implemented by their regional offices.

11 (2011): Eine Analyse der Versorgung psychisch Erkrankter (An analysis of the medical care of the mentally ill). Projektbericht „Psychische Gesundheit". Final report. p. 6.

In its „Analysis of the Care of Patients with Mental Illnesses", the Main Association of Austrian Social Security Institutions found that the average duration of annual sick leave caused by mental disorders is much higher than that caused by problems of physical health. The report of the study contains a detailed discussion of the inability to work due to mental problems.

See also the Salzburg regional health insurance body as well as GÖG/ÖBIG

See also: several studies have illustrated the dangers of this type of pressure to mental health, including those of the OECD (where nine countries were examined, Austria amongst them). In Austria, the Regional Public Health Insurance of Upper Austria, the Chamber of Labour of Upper Austria, pro mente Upper Austria and the pro mente academy had a closer look at this. According to a representative of the Regional Public Health Insurance, the main reason for retirement is mental illness. Every sixteenth day of sick leave is due to mental disorders.

See www.psychotherapie.at [10. 9. 2012].

See note of the OÖGKK. And: Decision-makers could exploite more this resource although the enormous potential for cost reductions in the health sector remains undisputed amongst experts.

12 Goldkinder (2007). Happy Princes (2011). Thomas Druyen, Dr. phil., sociologist and Director of the Institute for Wealthibility and Wealth Psychology at the Sigmund Freud University (SFU) in Vienna.

13 PthG, § 1. Kierein, Pritz, Sonneck. 1991. Psychologengesetz, Psychotherapiegesetz.
Kurzkommentar. 1991, p. 118.

14 See Elkington John and Hartigan Pamela (2008). In his introduction to this publication Klaus Schwab states that when the Schwab Foundation for Social Entrepreneurship (Klaus and Hilde Schwab) was founded in 1998 the term "social entrepreneurship" was still completely unfamiliar despite Ashoka's pioneer work in this area.

15 Achleitner et al (2007), p. 7. Achleitner holds the Foundation Chair on Entrepreneurial Finance at the Technical University in Munich, Germany.

16   The terms third sector, civil society, non-profit sector and similar are used as synonyms in this study.

17   Druyen Thomas (2007) Goldkinder. p. 60. Happy Princes (2011).

18   See also Bornstein David (2004); Bornstein is an American author who put five years of research into his book "How to change the world".

19   See Achleitner et al., 2007, p. 7.

20   See Dees, 1998/2001.

21   See Dees, 1998/2001, p. 1-2.

22   See also Linß, 2011.

23   Dees, 1998/2001, p. 4

24   Ibid. 2001, p. 1.

25   See www.ashoka.org.

26   Everyone a Changemaker, 2006, p. ii.

27   Drayton, See ibid.

28   Praszkier, Nowak and Zablocka-Bursa.Warsaw University. 2009, p. 42.

29   See also Mair & Martì, 2006; Stanford Center on Philanthropy & Civil Society u. a.; referring to „social", p. 37; article: Social Entrepreneurs Research, A source of explanation, prediction and delight.

30   2007. In: Social Entrepreneurship: The Case for Definition; Stanford Social Innovation Review.

31   See ibid. p. 35.

32   See www.grameen.org; (Grameenbank means village bank).

33   See Yunus, 2008, p. 34.

34   also anthropologist. Steps to an Ecology of Mind (1972)

Chapter 2

35   For the academically interested reader follows a brief description of the study:

The object of the study was the personality of the interviewed Social Entrepreneurs, their subjective attitudes, their way of thinking, how they feel and what environment they live in. The qualitative research methodology employed in the study was best suited for collecting the data needed, to describe and interpret them.

Significant criteria for a qualitative scientific analysis are the openness and flexibility of the researcher with regard to the questions asked, particularly in the case of unexpected new developments, contexts and results. The study is based primarily on personal interviews with social entrepreneurs in various countries of the world. In line with a data collection (methodology of *Grounded Theory* and a multidimensional research approach) it was ensured that a broad range of various interview partners was chosen, including some unusual ones (such as Muhammad Yunus).

With a specific combination of qualitative interview methods (including the narrative interview) and a respectful attitude, central aspects such as the core motivations of my interview partners could come to light without our discussions being restricted by rigid structures. In a next step the interviews were edited, evaluated and analysed.

36   See Interview # 1

37   Interview # 1, 78

38   Gloria de Souza was the 1st of Ashoka's Leading Social Entrepreneurs.

39   Interview # 2, 66 and 308

40   Interview # 3, 13

41   See Interview # 7,70

42   Interview # 5, 33

43   Interview # 5, 196

44   See Banker to the Poor, The Autobiography of Muhammad Yunus, Founder of Grameen Bank. 1998, mit Alan Jolis, Oxford University Press Ltd.

45   Interview # 6, 102

46   See Ashoka, Leading Social Entrepreneurs, 2009, p. 303; Interview # 6.

47   Interview # 11, 141

48   See 2001 and 2006, p. 29. (see also Conference on Resilience in Zürich in 2005) and see Hildebrand, 2006, p. 23.

49   See 3. World Congress of Psychotherapy. 2002.

50   Ist Charakter Schicksal? In: Profil (2012) No. 27, p.79. Authorisation to use the quoted text passage for this study received from the author. See also his publications "Persönlichkeitspsychologie" (2011) and "Psychologie der Persönlichkeit"(2012).

51   See Interview # 3

52   See Interview # 3

53   See Interview # 6, 17

54   See Interview # 5, 203

55   See Interview # 1, 84

56   See Interview # 2, 511

57   founded by Jeroo Billimoria; Aflatoun International offers social and financial education to millions

of children and young people worldwide empowering them to make a change for a more equitable world: www.aflatoun.org

Aflatoun International too was founded by Jeroo Billimoria. Aflatoun offers social and financial education to millions of children and young people worldwide empowering them to make a change for a more equitable world: www.aflatoun.org

See Interview # 4, 202

58   Social Entrepreneur, Founder and president of Lifegate; founder of Scaldasole, winner of awards www.lifeGate.it

See Interview # 9, 53: „Vivere con sentimento, dare un senso alla propria vita, consumare in un modo consapevole, rispettare l'ecosistema e tutte le forme di vita, cercare un lavoro gratificante, essere onesti con se stessi e con gli altri, fare del bene, scegliere vere amicizie, allontanare il dolore, la paura, la rabbia, vivere la vita con gioià, quindi questo sono i valori."

59   Interview # 9, 184. Scaldasole was the first biological company in Italy, founded by Marco Roveda in 1986. The social entrepreneur realised that it was not enough to work with the market only. So in 2000 the eco-cultural platform LifeGate was born which also consists of a network, a radio, a magazine and an internet portal to reach out to more people. [Original] "Ho trovato e ho capito che per essere felici dovremmo dare senso alla mia vita e dobbiamo fare del bene, dobbiamo essere gratificato e io ho trovato i valori che abbiamo

elencato prima. Capito questo, ho cominciato a vivere secondo questi valori e questi valori hanno condizionato la mia vita portandomi prima a fare fattoria Scaldasole, che è diventato l'azienda che ha creato il mercato del biologico in Italia. Quindi abbiamo diffuso valori di rispetto verso l'ambiente, verso le persone attraverso prodotti biologici." see also website www.lifeGate.it

60   Interview # 10, 46.

61   See Thomas Druyen (2012). Krieg der Scheinheiligkeit. Plädoyer für einen gesunden Menschenverstand: amongst others "Über Konkrethik", pp. 46-58.

62   Interviews # 2, 4

63   See Yunus, 1998.

64   "Performance work": this expression is used by others for his work as an artist (see documenta, Kassel, Germany). His father gave him a camera which has accompanied him since his youth. He describes it as "fundamental to my psychology."

65   [Original:] „Ho capito che per essere felici dovremmo dare senso alla mia vita e dobbiamo fare del bene."

66   Interview # 5, 107:

67   See origin. Friedrich Wilhelm Nietzsche: „Hat man sein Warum des Lebens, so verträgt man sich fast mit jedem Wie. [...]." See Frankl, 1973, p. 178; as well as the book chapter: "Der Aufgabencharakter des Lebens" www.viktor-franklschule.eu.

68   See 1990, p. 230.

69   See lecture notes, 2011, p. 8

70 Interview # 5, 514, 584 „Personal mission" refers to Youth Empowerment.

71 See 1996. Debats is psychotherapist and clinical psychologist

72 See Beck, 2012,

73 See Rieken's (2009, 2011) contribution to "mechanics" where he explains why mechanistic thinking was so successful. All physics as well as industrialization developed from it. However, profound changes are now underway in some areas (including quantum physics). The influence of mechanization was substantial throughout, in medicine and economics, too, and continues to have a great effect to this day. The effect of mechanistic thinking is dominant in some areas of psychology as well. Psychology emerged in an era of dispute between the approaches of natural sciences and humanities towards cognition. From the start psychology never was a uniform discipline. Psychoanalysis, too, has its mechanistic parts. For instance the id, ego and super ego is related, to some extent, to the structure of the brain. Freud wanted to be acknowledged by the natural sciences.

74 See Interview # 7, 58

75 2007, p. 68.

76 Interview # 2, 743

77 Interview # 3, 404:

78 Interview # 3, 247:

79 Interview # 6, 631

80 Interview # 9, 139; Original: "Questa base che è il bene [...] è il bene, fare del bene."

81 The list begins with an initiative in the health sector, as this study was undertaken within the framework of the health profession of psychotherapists. It is widely accepted that some phenomena are intermeshed, such as for instance poverty, social and cultural conflicts, health problems and education. Further, if ecology is under threat, this has an influence on all aspects of human life.

82 Interview # 6, 634, 295

83 Interview # 4, 204.

84 Rieken Bernd et al (2011). Publication series - psychotherapy sciences in research. Alfred Adler heute. Zur Aktualität der Indivdualpsychologie. Psychotherapiewissenschaft in Forschung, Profession und Kultur. Contributions: Joachim Prandstetter, Thomas Stephenson et al. Band 1. Waxmann pp. 207-219; Münster/New York/Munich/Berlin

85 My psychotherapeutic practice shows this is a reoccurring theme. The opposite of good is sometimes quoted as the well intended. Clients work through problems which have arisen due to misinterpretation of their good intentions. Or else they are suffering from personal harm caused by people in their social environment who had meant it well. To put it bluntly one could quote Jürgen Hargens (2007): "Please don't help! It is hard enough as it is." In specific situations caring professions are not exempt from this phenomenon. All parties involved need to reflect on this so that no harm is caused unvoluntarily to others through the act of helping.

86   Rieken et al (2011). Ibid # 84. Publication series - Psychotherapy sciences in research. Psychotherapiewissenschaft in Forschung, Profession und Kultur. Band 1. Waxmann; pp. 210-211; Münster/New York/Munich/Berlin

87   Goethe [1808]/1980, Verse 327-329, in Interview # 10.

88   Ibid. 474.

89   Interview # 6, 282.

90   See Interview # 5.

91   E.g. by speculating on food and state bankruptcies, through production processes in many parts of the world which are harmful to human health. See interviews with CEOs, brokers and others in the documentation.

92   See Summary and Outlook

93   Interview # 11, 9.

94   Interview # 2, 750: "[...] give your child the confidence to decide how he will discover himself, [...] so that's why I am in love with education."

95   See Interview # 3.

96   Interview # 5.

97   See Interview # 6.

98   Druyen. 2012. Verantwortung und Bewährung. Eine vermögenskulturelle Studie. p. 307.

99   See Austrian Psychotherapy Law (1990)

100   See Bateson, Satir, Haley, Selvini-Palazzoli, von Foerster, H. E. Richter, Merl, Stierlin, Simon, Duss-von Werdt, Welter-Enderlin u. a.: Sometimes this varies depending on the type of psychotherapeutic modality. The Systemic approach certainly

builds on the client's resources and potential for development.

Chapter 3

101   Interview # 1, 92: "But as I was in the village with the people I gratefully discovered the loan-sharks."

102   Interview # 5, 514

103   Ibid. # 584: "Many people have jobs they just hate and so it's a blessing to be able to live your life in service to your personal mission."

104   Interview # 7, 119.

105   Interview # 5, 20

106   See 2005. University of Pennsylvania

107   See the research social psychologists of Robert Emmons und Michael McCullough, Universities of California, Miami and Boston Research Center, 2010;

108   See www.bmg.gv.at:
        In systemic psychotherapy, for instance, interventions are implemented in structure constellations, if this is what the situation requires, to allow clients to experience acknowledgement. In this way people learn to value experiences differently. Information zum Themenbereich „Aufstellungsarbeit" in Psychotherapie und Beratung des Bundesministeriums für Gesundheit auf Grundlage eines Gutachtens des Psychotherapiebeirates [14. 6. 2005];

109   See Interview # 1 (Note: to help the poor to escape the debt trap.)

110 Opeka & Kansas, quoted in Welter-Enderlin, 2006, p. 11; See also the Chapter "Support – Honouring the Support Received" of this publication.

111 See 1992.

112 See 2006.

113 See 2006, S. 32.

114 See 2006, S. 20.

115 2002 [1991], Angelantonio Ferrandina. World Congress Psychotherapy 2002, Vienna. Director of I.A.M.S.; registered Mediator (Federal Justice Ministry), licenced Social and Life Counsellor, LifeCoach, Artist

116 Interview # 3, 324

117 2002 [1991], Angelantonio Ferrandina, ibid 115.

118 Interview # 3, 319

119 Interview # 7

120 See definition of cultural understanding, p.136

121 See Susanne Rippel, Christian Seipel. Methoden kulturvergleichender Sozialforschung. 2008.

122 See Interview # 3 and Interviews # 1, 2, 4.

123 See Interview # 3: The interview partner emphasised though that this can still work in the area of art. His personal explanation for this is that artists are deeply aware.

124 See Interview # 11.

125 See Interview # 10.

126 Interview # 7; "great neighbourhood" refers to the cultural context of where one grows up, to the peers as well as to professional contacts which were supportive in tackling the challenges as a social entrepreneur.

127 See Interview # 3.

128 Interview # 3, 583f.; the social entrepreneur is also active in the area of arts. His work has been shown at the well-known art exhibition "documenta" in Kassel, Germany as well as in India, Japan etc.

129 Works as an artist – both in the West (e.g. taking part at the documenta) and in the East (e.g. Japan)

130 See Interview # 3.

131 See 2006, S. 30.

131a www.journal-ethnologie.de [9. 2. 2011].

Chapter 4

132 See Angelantonio Ferrandina. (2015). Spirituality and Psychotherapy. World Journal Psychotherapy. #1 (8). pp.47-51.

133 Interview # 6, 49

134 Interview # 4

135 Interview # 3

136 Interview # 3. Work as an artist - in the West (e.g. taking part at the documenta) and in the East (e.g. Japan)

137 Interview # 5, 198

138 Interview # 1, 100

139 Interview # 1, 308

140 Interview # 7

141 Interview # 3

142 Ibid

143 also mediator and artist, founder and director of the training institution of counselling and mediation, I.A.M.S. Baden near Vienna; Austria. See

2002 [1991]. 3rd World Congress for Psychotherapy *anima mundi* in Vienna (2002);

144   See 2011, p. 8.

145   See also 2012

146   See Interview # 3.

147   See Goldkinder. 2007, p. 12. See ibid. Druyen. Schematic overview of the contents related to the concept of wealth. p. 12. Happy Princes. SFU. 2011 The Empowerment of wealthibility. SFU. 2011.

148   Interview # 1

149   Interview # 1, 111

150   Interview # 3, 84

151   Interview # 6, 110

152   Interview # 5, 29

153   See Interview # 3, 48.

154   See 2006, p. 7 See also Rieken, 2011, p. 207.

155   See 2006, p. 68.

156   Interview # 1, 336

157   Interview # 1, 291, 352 and Yunus, 2008, p. 157ff,

158   Interview # 6, 27

159   Interview # 2, 601, 620

160   Interview # 4, 94

161   Talk on the topic of social entrepreneurs by Bill Drayton in the Radiokulturhaus in Vinna on March 24, 2011 within the framework of the event series "Im Zeitraum" with Ö1 moderator Johannes Kaup.

162   Interview # 5, 489

163   Interview # 10, 328.

164   Interview # 2, 551

165 Interview # 3, 29, 478

166 Ibid.

167 See Roedig, Der Standard, 27. 10. 2012, ‚Great Spirit'.

168 See 2011.

169 See 2006, p. 67.

170 See 2003 and 1992.

171 See Walsh (2006)

172 Interview # 6, 143

173 Interview 11

174 See 2006.

175 Interview # 7, 34

176 The decision was taken to refrain from asking specific psychotherapeutic questions to gain more insight into that which remained unsaid. This decision was taken consciously. Anything else would have been unethical towards the personalities interviewed, as we agreed on an interview and not on a psychotherapeutic setting. See also the Austrian professional code for psychotherapists on www.bmg.gv.at: Bundesministerium für Gesundheit (2012). Berufskodex für Psychotherapeutinnen und Psychotherapeuten. Auf Grundlage von Gutachten des Psychotherapiebeirates, zuletzt vom 13. 03. 2012: Abteilung Rechtsangelegenheiten ÄrztInnen, Psychologie, Psychotherapie und Musiktherapie), paragraph VIII., p. 16.

177 Interview # 3, 273.

178 See also Interview # 7

179 See www.ashoka.org [29. 7. 2010] and E-Mail: 15. 1. 2015.

180   See Interview # 5

181   Interview # 6, 49

Chapter 5

182   See 2006, S. 35.

183   Supported by my experiences gained through many years of professional work as a mediator, social and life counsellor and psychotherapist.

184   For instance the argument "too big to fail" is sometimes used when referring to state interventions to save large banks and corporations.

Note within the context of personal responsibility: during a representative survey by the Austrian daily newspaper Der Standard in 2012 (See Oct 29, 2012, p. 7, Computer Assisted Telephone Interviews (CATI) representative for the Austrian population aged 16 and above, Oct 16 – 19, 2012) the participants were asked general and personal questions about justice, equality and fairness. The gist was: do you think there is justice in your country? Are you treated fairly or not really? Interestingly there was not a single question related to whether the participants had adopted an active role with regard to this topic. Nor was there any querying fair behaviour towards others. Personal responsibility seems to have low priority. A representative survey developed by a quality newspaper like The Standard (which often contains reflective contributions and analyses) can provide an indication of the general tendencies in society.

185   See Interview # 9

186 See Interview # 10 and E-Mail v. 15. 1. 2015.

187 See 2003b, 2006 S. 66

188 See Interview # 10.

189 See Interview # 1, Presentation at the Academy of Sciences, Vienna, May 28, 2009.

190 See Interview # 5.

191 Interview # 5

192 See 2006, p. 9.

193 See the public discussion of Muhammad Yunus and his daughter Monica Yunus, who is also a singer, on the topic of "social business and art" in the Museumsquartier in Vienna during the Global Social Business Summit, Nov 12, 2011. See also www.monicayunus.org and www.singforhope.org

Chapter 6

194 Original: Interview # 7

195 Original: Interview # 5, 9

196 Interview # 10.

197 Interview # 1, 145ff

198 Interview # 10 and E-Mail: 15. 1. 2015.

199 ibid.

200 See Monika Korber. What to do Now? Ethics in Psychotherapeutic Context. In: World Journal Psychotherapy (2015). # 1 (8) pp. 58-63

201 See also: For a deeper insight into mental structures: see Peter Dinzelbacher who illustrates the cultural history of mentality across several centuries (2003).

202 See 2006, p. 68.

203 See Murphy et al., 1974.

204 See Interview # 10.

205 Interview # 6, 653

206 Interview # 5, 131

207 See 2009. Drayton et al. Leading Social Entrepreneurs.

208 See Schober, Then et al.: Social Return on Investment. 2015; www.npo.or.at.
     See also: Ann-Christin Achleitner, Reinhard Pöllath and Erwin Stahl and co-authors have published concepts of financing and support for social entrepreneurs. Finanzierung von Sozialunternehmern. Konzepte zur finanziellen Unterstützungvon Social Entrepreneurs. 2007.

209 Thomas Druyen, 2011, p. 9; researcher on comparative wealth culture (wealthibility): "Vermögenskultur - Verantwortung im 21. Jahrhundert"

210 See well-known incidents of corruption, worldwide, in many parts of society;
     See TI: Transparency Internationawww.transparency.org; Global civil society organization fighting corruption.

211 Interview # 2

212 Interview # 5

Summary

213 Monika Korber, 2013.

214 Steve de Shazer and Insoo Kim Berg, Psychotherapists, Milwaukee Model.

215 See Angelantonio Ferrandina (2015). Spirituality and Psychotherapy. World Journal Psychotherapy. #1 (8) pp 47-51.

Outlook

216   The context of how theories developed and what effect they have on the individual and on society often don't receive enough attention, not only in economics. See also www.weltsozialforum.org; increasing global interest in social business

217   See EU-Study, ÖBIG as well as the Chapter "Introduction"

218   Compare the assessment of the Return on Investment (focused on material profit) with the assessment of the Social Return on Investment (SROI) with a focus on the benefit to society.

219   See Mary Gordon. – Roots of Empathy.

220   See WHO definition of health. See also chapters "Introduction" and "Questions of Meaning" in this book; See also EU-study on mental illnesses, an OECD study on job losses through mental pressures at the workplace amongst others (quoted in Der Standard of March 6, 2015)

Appendix

221   See Psychologie-Themenlexikon Geo, 2007, Bd. 13, p. 572.

222   Ibid.

223   See Asendorpf, 2010; Werner, 2005; Welter-Enderlin, 2006.

224   See dada-dada TV, 12. 10. 2011.

225   Ibid.

226   See Lamers-Winkelman, 2007, p. 45.

227   See EU-Study, 2012.

228   See Rieken, dada-dada TV, 12. 10. 2011.

229 Ibid. 2011.

230 See Themenlexikon Psychologie Geo, 2007, Bd. 13, p. 568.

231 Just like Schopenhauer before him Freud arrived at the same conclusion. 2006. Cordelia Schmid-Hellerau. Das Lesebuch. Schriften aus vier Jahrzehnten. [Original 1947]. Anna Freud. In: Gesammelte Werke. Eine Schwierigkeit der Psychoanalyse. Volume 12 (3-12)11.

232 See Rieken (2011a) (Ed). Alfred Adler heute. Zur Aktualität der Individualpsychologie. pp. 41-59, pp. 207-219.

233 See 2005. [Original 1963]. 14. Aufl. p. 241-270.

234 See Erik H. Erikson, 2005: Childhood and Society; Kindheit und Gesellschaft, p. 241ff.

235 Ibid.

236 Ibid. p. 243.

237 Initiators sometimes refer to their projects as "our/my baby".

238 See Erik H. Erikson, 2005: Childhood and Society.

239 See 2005 [Original 1963], p. 265.

240 Ibid. p. 266.

241 Ibid.

242 Ibid. p. 270-271, cursive original.

243 psychologist and researcher of psychotherapy, See 1989, p. 218.

244 See Duss-von Werdt, 2008, p. 24.

245 Chilean biologist, 1992, p. 32.

246 1994, p. 93.

247 The systemic psychotherapist Tom Levold wrote an overview of this. 2012, pp. 379-406

248 See Johnson, 1995. practitioner and lecturer in systemic psychotherapy

249 See the journal "Mensch und System", 1995.

250 Johnson, 1995, p. 8.

251 See Kuhl, 2001. University of Osnabrück

252 See 1990.

253 See 1997.

254 See Monika Korber (2015). What to do Now? Ethics in Psychotherapeutic Context. In: World Journal Psychotherapy. # 1 (8). pp. 58-63.

255 Druyen. Goldkinder. 2007, p. 180-187. Happy Princes. SFU. 2011

256 Antonovsky. Salutogenese. Zur Entmystifizierung von Gesundheit. 1997.

257 Ibid. p. 180.

258 Ibid. p. 181 and see systemic perspectives, including change of perspectives, connoting positively etc

259 See Bobbi Emel, 2011.

260 See Werner and Smith 1977, 1982, 1992, 2001, 2004, 2006.

261 ibid.

262 See Werner 2005

263 See 1987, 2000

264 See 1997

265 See also 2005, International Congress "Resilienz – Gedeihen trotz widriger Umstände".

266 See 1999 and 2012. Asendorpf is a researcher of the psychology of personalities.

267 See 1999

268 See 2006, p. 22-27. See Sociologist, Familytherapy;

269 See 2005, International Congress "Resilienz – Gedeihen trotz widriger Umstände".

270 Cited in Nuber, 2005, See APA, American Psychologist Association: In: The Road to Resilience.

271 2005.

272 Europe (Italy, Germany, Austria), Asia (India, Bangladesh), USA (Vermont, Massachusetts, Virginia).

273 Hannerz Ulf, 1992, Cultural Complexity. Studies in the Social Organization of Meaning. Psychiatric University Clinic (Psychiatrische Universitätsklinik) in Zürich, Switzerland, have developed transcultural psychiatry and psychotherapy at the university. Appadurai, 1996, Modernity at Large. Cultural Dimensions of Globalization. Wimmer Andreas (2005) Kultur als Prozess. Zur Dynamik des Aushandelns von Bedeutungen.

274 Schär Sall Heidi, Küchenhoff Bernhard, Schick Matthias (2011) Theorie und Praxis der transkulturellen Psychiatry and Psychotherapy at Psychiatric University Clinic Zürich. Unpublished manuscript made available by Ms Schär Sall.

275 Ibid. p. 2, 4.

276 Ibid.

277 See Luc Ciompi. Affektlogik, 2001, p. 15; and Ciompis lecture at SFU Vienna, 2006. Swiss psychiatrist

He was influenced, too, by Jean Piagets research results on the development of human mental structures and by Konrad Lorenz's work on the evolutionary roots of the mind.

278 Ibid., p. 17.

279 Ibid., p. 11.

280 See 2004, Lct., SFU.

281 See Luc Ciompi, 2001, p. 13.
Another consequence of ignorance within this context can be cynical forms of communication.
See ibid.; the psychiatrist Ciompi with his many years of professional experience notes with regard to the problems of psychotropic drugs: neuroleptics for instance have not nearly been researched sufficiently to really know what variety of effects they can have.

282 2009, Lct. SFU

283 See Gottfried Fischer, 2008, Logik der Psychotherapie and 2011. Psychotherapiewissenschaft. Einführung in eine neue humanwissenschaftliche Disziplin. Psychotherapist and psychologist at the University of Cologne, Germany.

284 See Fischer (1982) Handlungsvalidierung nach Wahl

285 See discussion of the Libet experiments, 1979; Fischer, 2008.

286 Ibid.

287 Fischer, 2008, 2011.

288 Event at the University of Vienna (2009). "The Final Crisis – The End of Globalization?" Note by Christian Felber (Attac – globalization-critical initiati-

ve) that for instance Keynes, too, was frequently misunderstood; Department of Economics, BA-CA Octogon Vienna on September 28, 2009; see also series of events at the Wirtschaftsuniversität WU-Vienna: Open Minds – "Sind wir alle Sozialdarwinisten? Das Menschenbild in der Ökonomie" with Helmut Schüller amongst others on June 16, 2009.

289 See Humberto Maturana, Congress, 1992, Die Wirklichkeit des Konstruktivismus, October 14 -18, 1992. Heidelberg.

290 Adam Smith, one of the classic economic thinkers from the time of pre-industrial capitalism, is often interpreted as follows: the actions of individuals, which are stimulated by self-interest, will lead to the benefit of the common good. (See Linß, 2011, p. 23ff.; from his popular work "An Inquiry into the Nature and Causes of the Wealth of Nations".) From a systemic perspective, however, hardly any consideration is given to the background to his theories, how and why they were developed, what the context was at the time and what their original intentions were. This would lead to a more differentiated interpretation.

291 See Crouch, 2009. British sociologist and political scientist

292 See Ciompi, 2001, p. 17.

293 See conference "Humanismus in der Medizin". Organiser: Innsbruck Medical University. Dept. for Clinical Nephrology [28.-30. 6. 2001].

294 See Ciompi, 2001

295 Profil No. 27, 2. 7. 2012; authorisation by the author (2012). Asendorpf received the Life-time Achievement Award of the European Association of Personality Psychology

The author participated at the following *theme-related events* (in chronological order):

IV (2008). Bewusst innovativ? – Society versus Technology. „Migration braucht Innovation?" Education, Innovation and Research. House of Industry.

Kernberg Otto (2008). „Die Persönlichkeit als Führungskraft." Heitger Consulting, Vienna Consulting Group. Vienna. 10. 11. 2008.

SFU (2008). „Erfolgsfaktor Freude – Soziale Gesundheit in Österreich." Working Group. Psyche & Economy. Vienna. 25. 11. 2008

SFU (2009). Conference „Osteuropäische versus Westeuropäische Mentalitäten: Gibt es Hoffnung auf ein gegenseitiges Verständnis?" Eastern versus Western European Mentalities – is there hope for mutual understanding?

Colin Crouch (2009). Speech „Post-Democracy". Österreichische Kontrollbank. Vienna. 5. 3. 2009.

MIT Europe Conference (2009). Schönbrunn. Vienna. 25. 3. 2009. Austrian Social Business Day (2009). Platform for CSR-Projects and Social Business. 21. 4. 2009.

SFU (2009). „Social Business Regionalkonferenz. Genisis going Vienna." Among others Thomas Druyen, Peter Spiegel, Andreas Idl u. a., SFU. Vienna. 14. 5. 2009.

Grüne Österreich (2009). „Über den Tellerrand ... Woher kam die Krise und wer holt uns da raus?" Alexander Van der Bellen and Willi Hemetsberger. House of Music. Vienna. 27. 5. 2009.

SFU (2009). Prof. M. Yunus. Austrian Academy of Sciences Vienna. 28. 5. 2009.

SFU (2009). „Westliche Couch und östliches Sitzkissen". Working Group – Transcultural research and Psychotherapy science: Head: Johannes Reichmayr, Christine Korischek. Wien. 26. 5., 16. 6. 2009.

Universität Wien (2009). "The Final Crisis – The End of Globalization?" BA-CA Oktogon. U. a. m. Christian Felber. Institut für Volkswirtschaftslehre, Vienna. 28. 9. 2009.

Vision Summit (2009). Social Business. "Another wall to fall." GENISIS. Institute for Social Business and Impact Strategies gemeinnützige GmbH. Free University Berlin. Berlin. 8. 11. 2009.

Ziegler Jean (2009). „Der Hass auf den Westen. Wie sich die armen Völker gegen den wirtschaftlichen Weltkrieg wehren." Volkstheater. Vienna. 25. 11. 2009.

Reemtsma Jan Philipp (2009). „Wie weitermachen mit Sigmund Freud? Anmutungen eines Nicht-Psychoanalytikers." Sigmund Freud Museum. Vienna. 10. 12. 2009.

Austrian Social Business Day (2010). Platform for CSR-Projects and Social Business. Vienna. 28. 2. 2010.

SFU (2010). International Conference „Psychotherapiewissenschaft und ihre Grundlagen". SFU. Vienna. 18.-19. 3. 2010.

IWM. Institut for Human Sciences (2010). Debating Europe. "Opportunities and Dangers of Immigration." Among others Speakers included Giuliano Amato. Kooperation der Standard und Erste Stiftung im Burgtheater. Vienna. 21. 3. 2010.

Vision Summit (2010). "Don't wait. Innovate! Generating Social & Business Innovators." GENISIS. Institute for Social Business and Impact Strategies gemeinnützige GmbH. University Potsdam. 8. - 9. 4. 2011.

ÖNB (2010). Emotional Capitalism. „The Market Frontier and Emotional Life." Arlie Hochschild, University of California, Berkley. Vienna. 8. 10. 2010.

WU (2010). „Open Minds" mit André Heller. Vienna. 20. 10. 2010. UBIT (2010). „Leadership 2020 – Werte & Wirtschaft". 8. Austrian IT & Beratertag Consultant Day. Imperial Palace. Speakers included Gerhard Schwarz, Herlmut Schüller. Vienna. 2. 12. 2010

Rifkins Jeremy (2011). Speech "Challenging Prospects – Rethinking Global Systems". Among others u.a.

Panelist. 8. Viennese Congress. Com.consult. Federation of Austrian Industries. Vienna. 25. 1. 2011.

NPO-Institut (2011). „Finanzierungsquellen in NPOs: Vielfalt als Strategie?" Kompetence Centre for Nonprofit Organisations. WU. Vienna. 15. 3. 2011.

Radiokulturhaus (2011). „Ökologie im Wandel. Social Entrepreneurs – Umwelt." Bill Drayton. 24. 3. 2011.

Vision Summit (2011). Don't wait. Innovate! Generating Social & Business Innovators. GENISIS. Institute for Social Business and Impact Strategies gemeinnützige GmbH. University Potsdam. Berlin. 8. - 9. 4. 2011.

SFU (2011). "Psychotherapy East & West: Contemporary Theoretical and Practical Perspectives." Vienna. 16.-20. 5. 2011.

RPP (2011). „Das Unbehagen mit der Religion. Institut für Religiosität in Psychiatrie und Psychotherapie." Institut für interkulturelle Islamforschung. SFU. Islamic Centre Vienna. 18. 6. 2011.

1. Kongress der transkulturellen Psychiatrie, Psychotherapie und Psychosomatik im deutschsprachigen Raum (2011). „Integration. Identität. Gesundheit." Alpen-Adria-University Klagenfurt. 23.-25. 9. 2011.

3rd Social Business Summit (2011). MQ and Ana Grand Hotel. Vienna. 9.-12. 11. 2011.

Radiokulturhaus (2012). „Warum wir kreative Visionen brauchen." Eurich Claus. Vienna. 15. 3. 2012.

Medical University Vienna, SFU, BÖP (2012). „Glück & Lebenszufriedenheit – Key Competence Happiness". Symposium. AKH. Vienna. 24. 2. 2012.

Arge Bildungsmanangement Wien (2012). V. Viennese Conference on Mediation. "Culture meets Culture" – Ubuntu and „Wie wir alle voneinander abhängig sind." Official Building of the Austrian Health Ministry. Vienna. 17.-19. 5. 2012.

Vierter Global Social Business Summit (2012). "Power of Innovation – To Change the World". Austria Center. Vienna. 8.-10. 11. 2012.

I.A.M.S. Mediationstagung. 12. 2. 2016. Albert Schweitzer Haus. Vienna

4gamechanger festival 2017. 22. – 25. 4. 2017. Vienna. Among others Forest Whitaker.

VI. Conference. Mediation und Gerechtigkeit. Mediation and Justice. 12. 5. 2017 Arge Bildungsmangement at SFU. Vienna.

Interviewpartners in alphabetical order:

Ravi Agarwal: Delhi, Chennai, India;
www.toxicslink.org www.raviagarwal.com

Jeroo Billimoria: Amsterdam, NL; Mumbai, India;
www.childline.org, www.aflatoun.org,
www.childfinanceinternational.org,
www.childhelplineinternational.org,

Bill Drayton: Arlington, Virginia, USA;
www.ashoka.org

Patricia Kahane: Vienna, Austria, Switzerland;
www.karlkahanefoundation.org

Judy Korn: Berlin, Germany;
www.violence-prevention-network.de

Rebecca Onie: Boston, Massachusetts, USA;
www.healthleads.usa.org

Earl Martin Phalen: Boston, Massachusetts, USA;
www.summeradvantage.org www.themindtrust.org

Marco Roveda: Merone, Italy; www.lifegate.it,
www.buenavistasocialgolf.org

Gloria de Souza: Mumbai, India; www.parisarasha.net;
Gloria de Souza peacefully passed away in 2013.

Alisa del Tufo: North Bennigton, Vermont, USA;
www.thresholdcollaborative.org www.connectnyc.org

Götz Werner: Karlsruhe, Germany;
www.unternimm-die-zukunft.de

Muhammad Yunus: Dhaka, Bangladesh; www.
grameenfoundation.org www.yunuscentre.org;
www.muhammadyunus.org

Further weblinks in alphabetical order: www.

activephilanthropy.org
aflatoun.org
architectsofthefuture.net
ashoka.org
aspeninstitute.org

betterplace.org
bonventure.de
bmg.gv.at http://bmg.gv.at/cms/home/attache-
ments/6/8/3/CH1002/CMS1144348592 885/berufsko-
dex.pdf): Berufskodex für Psychotherapeutinnen und
Psychotherapeuten
buenavistasocialgolf.org
bus.ualberta.ca/ccse

changemakers.net
childline.org
childfinanceinternational.org
childhelplineinternational.org
concrethics.com
connectnyc.org
cropster.org

ecofriends.com
eine-welt-handel.at
erstestiftung.org
esslsozialpreis.at
europsyche.org/download/cms/100510/EAP_ethical_
guidelines.pdf

fairix.de
foursome.net

gexsi.org
glocalist.com; http://betauser.glocalist.de
gsbs2012.com
gute-tat.de

healthleads.usa.org

idealist.org

jugendeinewelt.at

ksghauser.harvard.edu
karlkahanefoundation.org
kinderzentren.de
krieg-der-scheinheiligkeit.de
kspope.com/ethcodes/index.php

leadertoleader.org

mckinsey.com/clientservice/nonprofit/hompe.asp
muhammadyunus.org

newenergies.ch/index_di.html
npo.or.at

oikos-international.org
oneworld.net

parisarasha.net
planethelp.de

rainbows.at
raviagarwal.com
riseproject.org

schwabfound.org
sfu.ac.at
skollfoundation.org
socialbusinessday.org
socialedge.org
socialimpactaward.at
sozialbank.de
sozialmarie.org
stiftungen.org
streetfootballworld.org
summeradvantage.org
street-uk.com

the-hub.net
themindtrust.org
thresholdcollaborative.org
toxicslink.org
triodos.de

ubit.at
unternimm-die-zukunft.de
utopia.de

violence-prevention-network.de

waldzell.org youthventure.org

yunuscentre.org

Film documentations

In certain aspects the film documentations contribute to a better understanding of the researched phenomenon. (See research principle of David Rennie, University Toronto)

Achbar Mark, Abbott Jenifer, Bakan Joel (2004). The Corporation. The pathological pursuit of profit and power. Sundance Festival.

Bonsai People. The Vision of Muhammad Yunus. A Documentary by Holly Mosher. BonsaiMovie.com (Screening, 8. 11. 2011. Grand Hotel, Wien).

Ferguson Charles (2010). Inside Job. Film Festival Cannes, Toronto, Telluride, New York.

Goeres Achim (2010). Chaos – Höllenfahrt zur Transformation. Calumed-Kongress. Chaos. Schöpfung. Evolution. Bispingen.

Hofmann Albert (1998). Insights and Outlooks. AV Record. Roge. Kaufen für die Müllhalde: http://tinyurl.com/solfilm-muellhalde. Ndumbe III Kum'a (2008). Identitäten zwischen den Welten. Calumed-Kongress.

Sauper Hubert (2004). Darwin's Nightmare. Eine Reise in das Herz Afrikas und das Innere des globalen Wirtschaftssystems. Falter: Wien.

Senf Bernd (2008) Globalisierung, Börsenfieber und
kollektiver Wahn. Calumed- Kongress: Globalisierung
und Identität. Berlin.

Wagenhofer Erwin (2008). Let's make money. Delphi:
Berlin.

Abbreviations

a. o.	among others
Art.	Article
BMG	Federal Health Ministry – Bundesministerium für Gesundheit.
EAP	European Association of Psychotherapists
GSBS	Global Social Business Summit
GT	Grounded Theories
NAI	Narrative Interview
NPO	Non Profit Organisation
ORF	Österreichischer Rundfunk – Austrian Broadcasting Corporation
QI	Qualitative Interview
PthG	Psychotherapy Law (Austria)
ROI	Return of Investment
p.	page
SFU	Sigmund Freud University
SROI	Social Return of Investment
TI	Transparency International
TU, Vienna	Technical University